yoga

with your child

yoga

with your child

150 yoga moves to enjoy together

Alice Lageat & Béatrice Raphalen

Illustrated by Youlie

GREEN TREE

LONDON • OXFORD • NEW YORK • NEW DELHI • SYDNEY

GREEN TREE
Bloomsbury Publishing Plc
50 Bedford Square, London, WC1B 3DP, UK
29 Earlsfort Terrace, Dublin 2, Ireland

BLOOMSBURY, GREEN TREE and the Green Tree logo are trademarks
of Bloomsbury Publishing Plc

First published in 2020 in France as *Yoga avec son enfant* © 2020, Editions First,
an imprint of Edi8, Paris, France

First published in Great Britain 2022

A catalogue record for this book is available from the British Library

Library of Congress Cataloguing-in-Publication data has been applied for

ISBN: TPB: 978-1-4729-9278-9

2 4 6 8 10 9 7 5 3 1

Typeset in Santral Light
Printed and bound in India by Replika Press Pvt. Ltd.

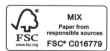

To find out more about our authors and books visit www.bloomsbury.com
and sign up for our newsletters

Contents

Foreword by Sophie d'Olce 7

Introduction 9

Ten good reasons to practise yoga
with your child 11

Why yoga and how to practise 13

Sequences

An introduction to the joints of your body 37

Sun salutation 45

The cat 53

The koala 63

The strange magic machine 75

The butterfly 91

A walk by the pond 103

The fairy 121

The elephant 141

The duck 155

The grasshopper 173

The camel 189

The flamingo's day 207

Warrior training 221

The monkey 233

Index 249

Foreword by Sophie d'Olce

Artistic Director of Compagnie Maya, organisers of various parent–child workshops (baby signing, dance, theatre, yoga) www.compagniemaya.com

For most parents, daily life is a roundabout – a never-ending list of logistical and organisational constraints. This frenetic pace, where time flies by and we struggle to keep up, doesn't really fit with what we actually want from life with our children. Getting away from the daily routine in order to do what we really want is not always easy, but a parent–child activity can be the ideal way to take a break.

In the workshops we hold at Compagnie Maya we believe that taking part together lets us transport ourselves to a special time and place, to our own bubble outside 'normal' time: a healing place, somewhere to (re)connect with the present moment. We spend time with our child; we tell them how happy we are to be here with them and how special they are.

To share an experience, to discover a discipline that is new to both parties, puts the parent and the child on the same level. The hierarchy has gone; the parent does what the child does and is not simply a spectator or a companion. The parent participates in the activity as a student, on exactly the same level as the child.

It is rare to do this in Western society, where we have the tendency to keep everything separate: activities for adults on one side and those for children on the other. And in our culture it is not always easy for an adult (who perhaps isn't used to this type of activity) to place themselves in an unknown situation, in (relative) discomfort, and to take (small) risks.

This way of practising allows us to (re)discover each other in a different context, outside daily life, and look at each another with fresh eyes. Learning new things together is conducive to laughter and, above all, sharing. Parent and child are complicit, united in play and the pleasure of doing things together. Taking part in activities together encourages the parent–child bond, and strengthens the relationship and the love.

Introduction

Practising yoga with your child lets you take part, at home or away from it, in an activity that is both athletic and relaxing, and that will enrich and reinforce the parent–child relationship. Fundamental to it is an awareness of the body, of breathing and of relaxation. The different sequences are fun and varied, and suitable for both parents and children. Throughout the 15 yoga sequences, the breathing exercises, the relaxation and the meditation, this book is designed to be a simple, interactive tool that allows you to enjoy some special time together, undertaking activities where parent and child do the same thing at the same time.

Whether you are beginners or experienced participants, this book is for parents who want to help their children discover yoga. The yoga sequences are designed for children aged four to ten years old, and are also suitable for mums and dads. Practice is as beneficial for the little ones as it is for the big ones! Certain sessions are more suited to those with more experience[1] and this is indicated at the beginning of each set, but the moment you start it is important, for you as a parent, as well as for your child, to do only what you are comfortable with, and to improve slowly but surely as you practise.

By learning and practising yoga together with that in mind, you have the chance to demonstrate, and thereby pass on to your child, certain valuable qualities, such as humility, perseverance and even patience. By showing them your determination and your concentration, as well as your ability to let go, your child will follow your example and also see you in a different light. It's a fun and

---

[1] In France a 'yogist' is someone who practises yoga. A yogi is someone who dedicates their entire life to yoga, through practise as well as their daily actions, their way of life and their behaviour, all of which is consciously performed with the philosophy of yoga in mind. In this book, as is common in the English language, we use 'yogi' to describe what the French refer to as a yogist.

practical way to demonstrate those values and qualities, rather than just talking about them.

By starting this new activity, you will create a new channel of communication beyond words. It is passed on through the physical, through mutual learning, with sharing and kindness. Practising the poses, breathing exercises, relaxation and meditation in a pair gives you the chance to discover your body, your mobility and new possibilities, and also gives you access to part of a new inner life. You will feel the liberation of certain emotions and mental stimulation thanks to the increased concentration needed to practise yoga.

Practising yoga with your child will give you the opportunity to create a special time and place in which you are totally available to share the moment with them, and to listen to them as you work together.

So let's get started in this new adventure. It will be a huge source of pleasure for both you and your child!

Ten good reasons to practise yoga with your child

1
Develops your parent–child bonding through
a new experience

2
Allows you to learn more about each other while
doing the same activity together

3
Helps with body and breathing awareness
from a very young age

4
Gives access to an array of simple techniques to
aid rest, healing and relaxation

5
You are there for your child and share
a truly unique moment

6
Creates a listening space for yourself and your child

7
Enables you to take some time out from the world

8
Allows you to see each other in new light

9
Strengthens the rapport you have with your child

10
Creates some wonderful memories

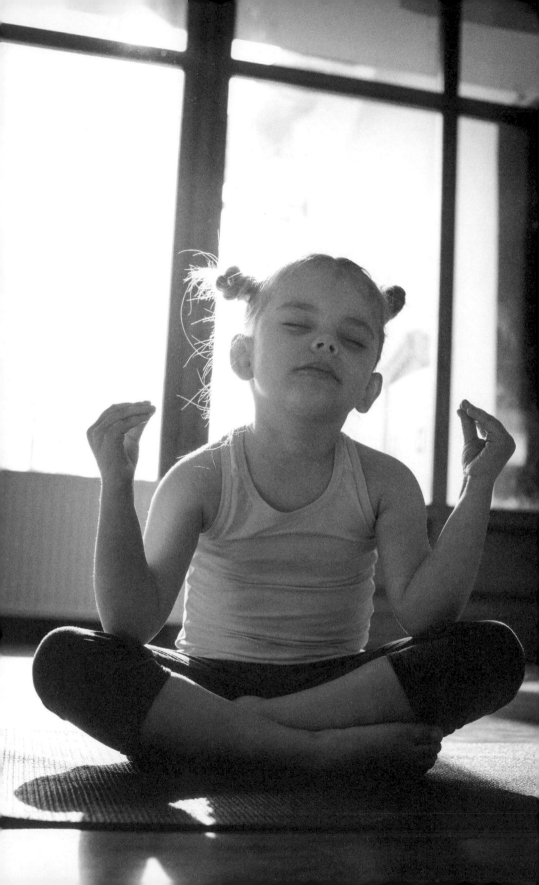

Why yoga and how to practise?

In this section we answer your questions about the origins and practice of yoga.

What does 'yoga' mean?

In the workshops we run the meaning of the word yoga is one of the most commonly asked questions and it's asked as much by parents as by children.

Yoga is a Sanskirt (ancient Indian language) word, it's root 'yog' means to attach or join.

Yoga is the union of the individual consciousness with the infinite consciousness; the union of earth and skies; the union of the individual and the universal.

Yoga also allows the union of different parts of a person, particularly the physical body, the mind and the emotions and that union goes beyond the internal and external, creating harmony between the human being and the outside world.

Yoga is a practice that, by its very essence, creates a link, and one of the intentions of this book is to encourage that link between parent and child.

More generally, yoga is a comprehensive approach that uses a number of specific techniques related to Indian traditions.

What does yoga consist of?

The practice of yoga is made up of many different elements and encompasses a series of varied exercises. It could be poses or movements (called 'asanas' in Sanskrit) that take place on a yoga mat, or some meditation, time spent concentrating on your breathing, chanting a mantra, or having a respectful and benevolent attitude towards yourself and others. Yoga allows us to find balance in all aspects of our lives, as the master yogis do. Yoga does demand concentration and rigour, but after a yoga session you can often feel as light as a feather.

Yoga can give us progressive awareness of the various elements of ourselves – our body, mind and spirit – and by practising the poses, breathing and relaxation we can improve our overall well-being.

What are the effects of yoga?

The benefits of yoga are common to both children and adults.

Yoga helps us to heal. Spending time on it enables us to relax. Yoga is practised in a relaxed manner, while fully conscious of body and breath, and it helps us improve our well-being and encourages healing.

Yoga helps us to increase our concentration and attention. The practice also helps channel our energy and regulate our emotions.

Yoga is not a competitive activity. On the contrary, each person does what they can and improves at their own pace, not in comparison to others. Even great yogis are constantly evolving and have room for improvement. Through yoga we seek comfort and stability, and progressively find balance in the poses and breathing. This balance brings a positive and conscious feeling in the body, and it becomes our ally. We also realise the value of the link between mind and body, and the joy such activity brings us with respect to body and consciousness. It also allows us to learn total humility, perseverance and patience. In yoga there is no failure, just constant learning. Thanks to these virtues, yoga helps with our self-confidence and self-esteem. Slowly but surely, as we practise, we improve; we are better connected to ourselves, but also to other people and the outside world; we have more space in our bodies and more lightness of breath. We also become more at ease with new life experiences.

Practising yoga is also an opportunity to discover your body in a different way. To feel, listen to and respect it. It opens up a limitless exploration of our motor skills from the youngest age. Our mobility is encouraged and improved, awareness of the position of our body is constantly stimulated and that helps enormously in our daily lives.

Through practising yoga we can gently improve our breathing, flexibility and muscle strength. We progress gradually and without pressure to find ourselves in a better place physically: there is less tension in the body, we have improved digestion, we find it easier to relax and we experience a calmness of mind.

Thanks to the framework that is put in place by learning yoga, we are able to let go in a way that is extremely beneficial to our own personal fulfilment.

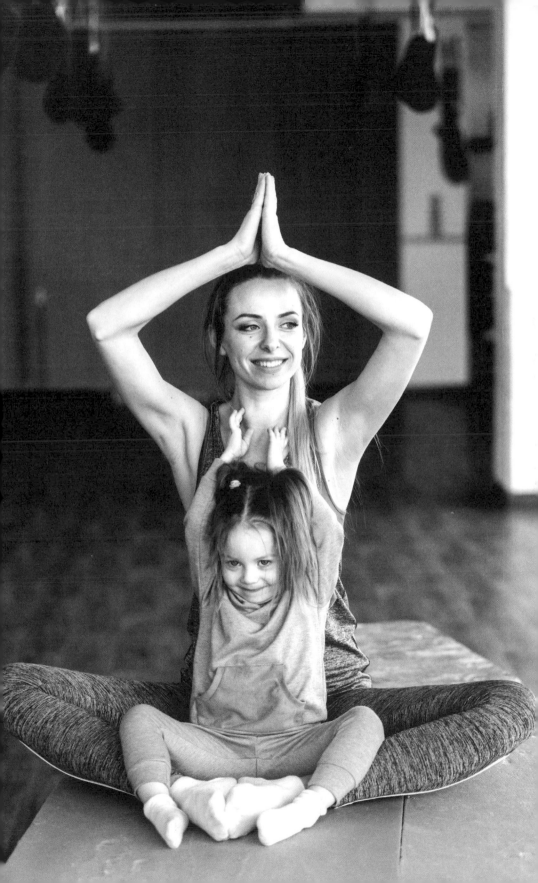

A yoga session at home

As you would in a yoga class, we suggest that at home you organise your session with your child in the following way:

1. Set up your space

2. Start the session in yogi pose, chanting the om mantra

3. Carry out the sequence of poses

4. Relax

5. Meditate

6. End the session in yogi pose, chanting the om mantra

7. Tidy up your space

Note these steps, as well as the breathing that goes with them throughout each session.

We recommend that you practise yoga on an empty stomach, at least two hours after a meal or in the morning before breakfast.

Create a space where you will do yoga

The intention of this book is to help you enjoy special time with your child while you do yoga. Organising a physical space contributes to creating this special time. Yoga is a discipline that requires concentration: the right environment and a willingness to focus are important in order to reap its benefits fully. For the former, choose a place in your living area with enough space to be able to move around freely. It should be clean, calm and well ventilated, and ideally not too cluttered so you won't be distracted. If the weather is fine you can go outside, but not into direct sunlight. Arrange your accessories – a mat each, cushions if you think you might need them and a blanket each – and have a little water to hand.

Create a warm ambience with low-level lighting.

If you like, you can also make a small shrine. You and your child can choose an object or an image that means a lot to you and encourages contemplation.

As you set up the space you are beginning your yoga session, creating a peaceful space in your daily life where you can unwind.

Yogi pose

Throughout this book we often ask you to get into yogi pose, also known as easy pose or 'sukhasana' in Sanskrit. This pose is an anchor for the start of the sequence: we set up this way when we begin practice. A yogi notes what is there in the present moment and that they are present in their body. Even while meditating and seemingly doing nothing, they are present and this begins with their way of sitting.

To get into yogi pose, sit cross-legged with your sit bones well anchored on the floor, your back and the top of your head up straight, looking directly ahead of you. Place your hands on your knees, your palms facing upwards, shoulders relaxed. Imagine you are a puppet held up by a thread that is attached to the top of your head. In order to keep your back straight, visualise

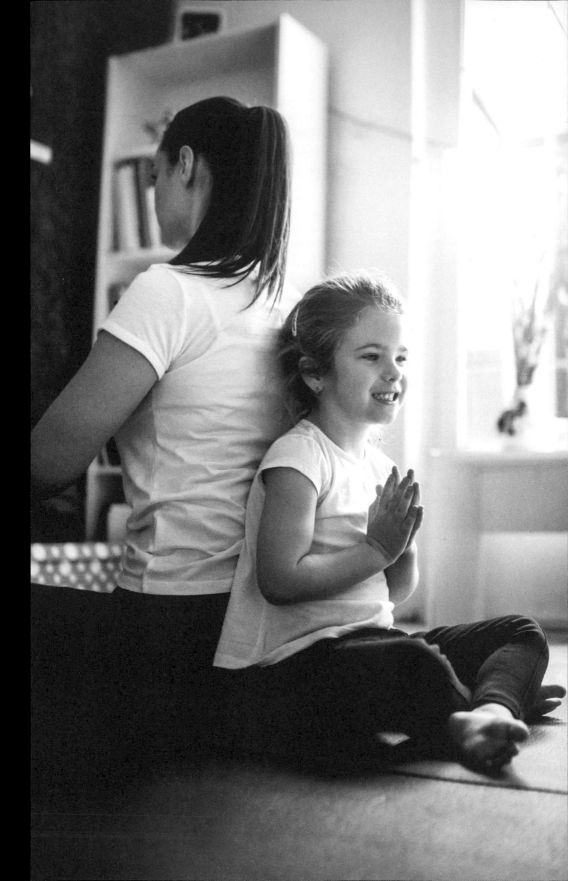

somebody checking the whole of your back. Try to align the back of your skull with a line down to your sacrum (the bone between your buttocks). You may need to tuck your chin in slightly. Muscles should be tensed, but not tight.

Om: the mantra for starting and ending

A yoga session begins with the chanting of a mantra. Like lighting a candle, this signifies the start of the session. Many different types of mantra can be chanted at the start. The most common is the sound 'om', which is widely considered to be the original sound, the primordial sound in the yoga universe. The om sound contains all that has been, is and will be. It incorporates all that we are and all that surrounds us.

The om sound includes all the sounds in the universe and, more precisely, the three sounds ah–oo–mm. Going around these three sounds, we take a journey through the entire cycle of life. The ah is for the beginning, the oo is the duration and continuity, and the mm represents the end – destruction with the possibility of renewal. The silence that follows the sound is as important as the part that is chanted.

Om has a strong vibration to it, so you can feel it if you chant it. There are a number of mental, physical and spiritual advantages to chanting om, and a number of scientific studies have proved the health benefits of doing so.

Both of you should sit face to face in the yogi pose, with your hands together as if in prayer, your thumbs level with your sternum and your forearms parallel with the floor. You can close your eyes to feel more present and to fully feel the effects of the mantra.

Take three deep breaths, as explained on page 26, and then breathe deeply in through your nose, lips slightly open, and breathe out slowly, letting your vocal chords vibrate with the 'ah-oo' sound until your lungs are totally empty. To make sure the sound is the right one you can put your hand flat on your thorax (sternum), level with your collarbone, or on your child's, so you can feel the vibrations.

When the breath feels fully exhaled, close your mouth and pull in your stomach to expel the rest of the air while making the 'mm' sound. This will resonate in your skull.

Chant three times. Feel the vibration and encourage your child to feel it, too.

Children may find this strange the first few times they do it. Sometimes it makes them laugh a lot. If you feel it's necessary, take the time to practise in a more formal manner.

The chanting of the mantra at the start of a session is a great way of conditioning yourself. By chanting om three times we focus fully on our breathing and we concentrate on the present moment. The vibrations that we feel serve to wake up our bodies, give us an awareness of our inner selves and encourage us to concentrate. Also, the vibrations that come from chanting the om mantra help to relax us, like a form of lullaby, setting us on the path to calmness and full consciousness.

There are many mantras used to finish a yoga session. We suggest you end your practice with the same mantra you started it with, chanted three times while sitting in the yogi pose, with your hands together in prayer in front of your sternum.

Breathing

Of the many elements that make up yoga, breathing is one of the most important. We use deep breathing, through the nose, and it is essential to use it throughout the entire session. Breathing is the basis of life. Because of the movement of the diaphragm, the main muscle associated with breathing, our ribs move from the very first day of our lives to our last. In the first few years of our lives, when we are babies, we breathe in this way, from the belly. We learn to do this again through yoga.

Working on your breathing is not easy and often, as adults, we breathe with our mouths and our upper bodies. Thanks to this practice, however, parents as well as children will adopt better habits and re-educate their breathing. Once a child has adopted this practice it will be with them for life!

Correct breathing posture is very powerful. It allows you to stay calm, to concentrate, to appease your anger and to calm your fears. Breathing correctly can help us grow, stay healthy, stay supple and also give us more energy when we need it.

In yoga there are many different types of breathing. We have decided to go into detail on traditional breathing and long, deep breathing, whether you are sitting or lying down. Long, deep breathing is similar to traditional breathing, but it follows a slower rhythm and longer exhalations. Other types of breathing are looked at in certain sequences, for specific needs.

Yoga breathing is done through the nose with your mouth closed. Put your lips together, but don't clench your teeth. Rest your tongue gently on the roof of your mouth. As you breathe in, your belly expands to let in the air, right to the bottom. As you exhale, the belly goes back towards the spine, as if pushing all the air from your body.

To help your child understand, try asking them this riddle: 'What is your mouth for?' Your child will reply with something like: 'Talking! Eating!' Then ask them: 'What is your nose for?' They will probably say: 'Smelling, breathing, snoring!' You can then explain that in yoga we breathe through the nose because the mouth is made for talking, eating and yawning, but not breathing!

From a physiological point of view, breathing through the nose is better than through the mouth as it allows better oxygen transfer, and the nose better filters and moistens the air.

Long, deep breaths

In order to better understand breathing, you could try this exercise with your child. Get them to lie down on their back. Place a stuffed animal, a light toy or simply your hand on their belly. Ask your child to breathe in slowly through the nose, inflating their tummy as much as possible. Your child will be able to see the object rising up on the hill formed by their stomach. Then ask them to breathe slowly out through the nose and let the tummy go down. They will see the toy descend as well.

A breath in followed by a breath out makes one full breathing cycle. By simply breathing slowly and deeply your child will see their toy go up and down.

You can let your child have a go by telling them to put an object on your belly and making sure that you do the movement correctly.

To take this a step further – depending on the age of your child and their level of understanding – explain to them that a long, deep breath has three phases:

- First, the abdomen fills.
- Then, the ribcage opens and fills up.
- Finally, air gets into the upper part of the lungs, right up to your collarbones, which has the added effect of opening out your shoulders.

This order is for when you breathe in and it's the reverse for when you breathe out. Experiment and try out the three phases with your child.

Classic breathing while sitting

While sitting in yogi pose, tell your child to place one hand on their belly and, without blocking it, the other hand under their nose.

Explain to your child that when they breathe in, with the hand that's resting on it they will feel their stomach inflating, but they won't feel anything on the hand under their nose. And when they breathe out, they will feel their belly going in and, on the hand that's under their nose, they will feel the air coming out of their nose.

Once you have done this, sit facing each other and each place one of your hands on your stomach and the other on your ribcage at sternum level. As you breathe in, your belly inflates first, then your ribcage fills up to your collarbone. As you breathe out, first the air leaves from your collarbone area, then your ribcage deflates and finally your stomach, as your belly button moves gently towards your spine.

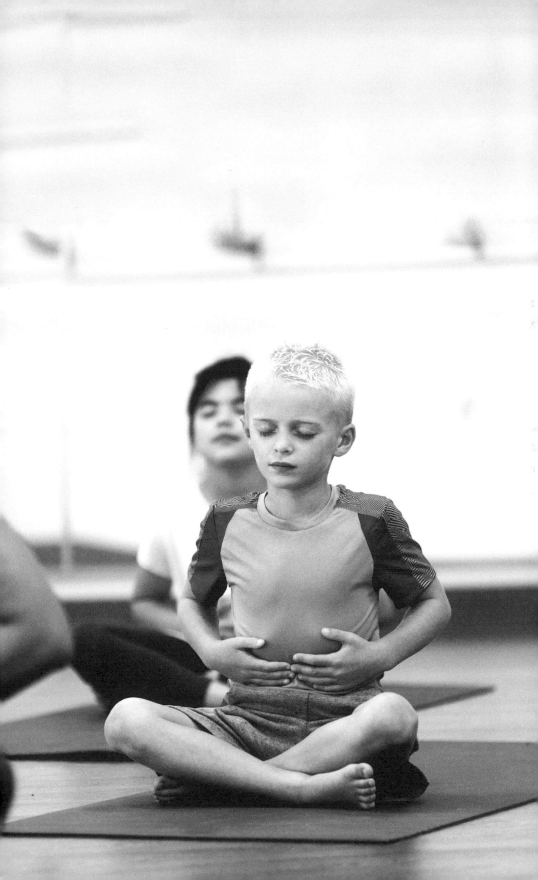

Relaxation

Relaxation is a key part of yoga. It is undertaken at the end of a session, before chanting a mantra. In each of our sessions, relaxation is shown by this feather:

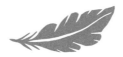

Adapt the length of your relaxation to the length of the session. For the shortest sessions you could try 10 minutes or so, but for the longer ones feel free to try a relaxation period more like 15 or 20 minutes.

In order to relax, lie on your back, arms and legs spread so your body is as loose as possible, palms upwards. You could lie next to each other. This could also be a good time to try your deep breathing techniques, but if your child chooses this moment for a big cuddle, that's also fine!

If you like, you could also try relaxation with yoga nidra. This practice consciously puts you into a state of deep relaxation (another way of describing it is 'lucid sleeping'). The process is a sort of body scanning in which you slowly and deeply visualise each part of the body, and it lets you access a state of complete relaxation while staying fully conscious.

Yoga nidra is done lying down, arms and legs gently spread so you are fully relaxed. Palms are turned up to the sky, eyes closed.

Your child lies like this and you sit in yogi pose, on a cushion if you wish. When both of you are ready, in a low voice, calmly and clearly, pausing regularly, read the text below:

'I am aware of myself lying on the floor. I can feel the whole length of my body against the floor. My head is relaxed. I can feel the back of my head against the floor. I can feel my skull and my scalp. My skull is relaxed. I can feel my face, my forehead, my nose, my eyes, my cheeks, my jaw, the inside of my mouth, my tongue, my chin. My face is relaxed. The whole of my head is relaxed. I can feel the front of my neck and the back of my neck, the muscles between my neck and my shoulders. I can feel my shoulders, my collarbone and my shoulder blades. My neck and my shoulders are relaxed. I can feel my arms resting on the floor. I can feel my elbows, my wrists, my hands and each one of my fingers. My arms are relaxed. I can feel my ribcage. I can visualise each one of my ribs as they move slowly with the rhythm of my breathing. My breastbone is relaxed. I can feel my diaphragm moving gently. My ribcage is relaxed. I can feel my stomach. I can feel my intestines, which are being slowly massaged by the movement of my breathing. I can feel my belly go up and down with the rhythm of my breathing. My stomach is relaxed. I can feel my pelvis, my hips, my buttocks, and the end of my spine on the mat, and it feels like it's getting slowly heavier. My pelvis, the area between my hips, is relaxed. I can feel my legs, my thighs, my knees, my calves and my ankles. My legs are relaxed. I can feel my feet, the arches of my feet, my toes. My feet are relaxed.

I am spread out and loose on the floor. My entire body is relaxed. I am listening to my breathing, which is deep and calm, and washing over my chest like a wave.

I am relaxed.'

Once you have read this, let your child breathe in and out a few times, and ask them to roll on to one side and then, with their eyes still shut, sit up in yogi pose. They can then open their eyes in order to end this yoga nidra practice.

Once you have done this a few times your child may well be able to have a go at guiding you in this relaxation – make the most of it!

Meditation

Meditation is an age-old practice, used in the East by Buddhists as well as by Ancient Greeks in the West. Today, after many studies, the benefits of meditation are recognised by scientists.

The goal of meditation is to observe and increase awareness of what we really are, our true nature, without judgement. This will lead us to go beyond our usual perceptions and beliefs.

In order to do this, we have to use our attention as a tool. We are going to focus our attention mainly on our breathing.

Meditation has numerous benefits. It allows us to listen to what we are really feeling and to recognise our emotions, to express them and to welcome them. In this way, we may understand our emotions better and, if necessary, transcend our feelings about the situation that caused those emotions.

Meditation will help calm our stronger emotions and manage stress. Practised regularly, it can aid concentration.

By introducing our children to meditation we are giving them a useful tool that they will be able to use themselves if they should need to.

You can meditate before going to bed in order to help you get to sleep.

By meditating we get in touch with our inner silence, which allows us to see clearly and make the right decisions.

Meditation encourages us to really listen to ourselves, which also helps us to listen to others.

There are many ways to meditate. It could be in silence, guided by a teacher whose voice you follow, or even while moving, or chanting mantras, or both.

Meditation with your child could be done at the end of a yoga session after the relaxation or at any time of day, whenever it suits your child.

Meditating before going to bed can help your child calm themselves down and may also help them get rid of high levels of emotion that they may have accumulated during the day, which will help them get to sleep.

You could also encourage your child to meditate if they feel sad or angry, in order to calm them down, or before a test or competition, in order to help manage any stress and encourage self-confidence.

To help you try out meditation with your child, we have a simple way of practising at home. Sit in yogi pose, hands on your knees, palms upwards and shoulders relaxed. Close your eyes. For parents and children who are used to meditating, you could focus your concentration on the point between your eyebrows, the 'third eye' or 'ajna' in Sanskrit, which encourages pineal gland activity (the pineal gland regulates the body's daily rhythms).

Concentrate on keeping your breathing steady and, without changing it, simply observe your breath as it goes in and out.

According to the NSF (National Science Foundation), we have around 30,000 thoughts a day, or about one thought every three seconds, so if thoughts spring into your head while you meditate, don't feel guilty; let them come and let them go like a passing cloud, without distracting you, and concentrate again on your breathing.

For young ones it is more difficult to maintain concentration for a long time. If your child is able to meditate even for five to 15 seconds, that's a lot! Congratulate them and encourage them. They will gain self-confidence and benefit without it becoming a chore. They will enjoy meditating on a regular basis, and will be able to improve the length and number of times they do it. It can become a very useful resource.

Above all, do not force them, as this will have the opposite effect. Our intention is to enjoy some fun moments together and feel the benefits.

In order to get your child used to meditation you can also sound a bell or a Tibetan bowl – something gentle – and encourage your child to concentrate on the way the sound is loud at the beginning, but fades until it disappears completely.

Yoga sequences for two people

We have created 15 different sequences, divided by age, length of session, time of day and difficulty level.

The 15-minute sessions are the easiest:

- An introduction to the joints of your body
- Sun salutation
- The cat
- The koala

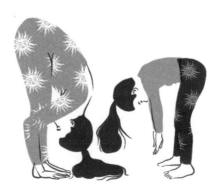

The 15- to 30-minute sessions are a bit more difficult:

- The strange magic machine
- The butterfly
- A walk by the pond
- The fairy
- The elephant
- The duck
- The grasshopper

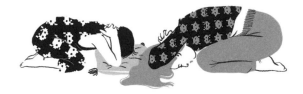

The 20- to 30-minute sessions are the most difficult:

- The camel
- The flamingo's day
- Warrior training
- The monkey

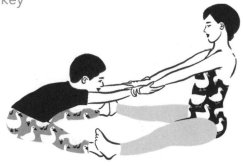

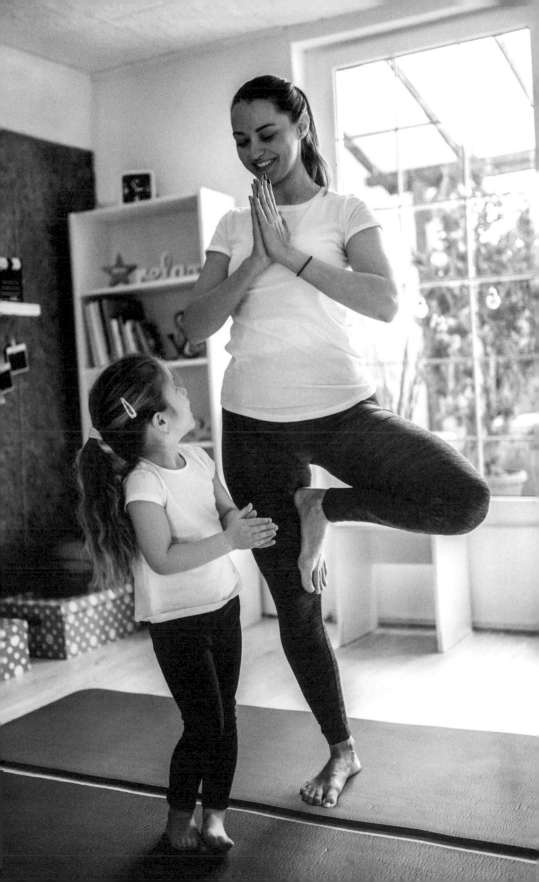

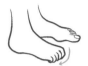

1. Toes

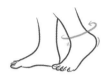

2. Ankles

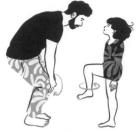

3. Knees

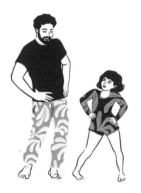

4. Pelvis

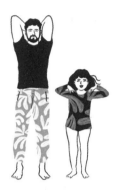

5. Shoulders

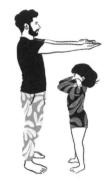

6. Elbows

7. Wrists

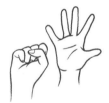

8. Fingers

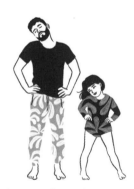

9. Neck

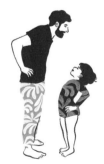

10. Upper back

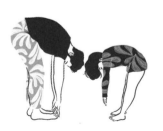

11. Lower back

An introduction to the joints of your body

For all ages
For all levels – perfect for beginners
For any time of day
Duration: 5 to 15 minutes

This session enables you to learn about the various joints in the body and to get them moving. This is a good one for the morning as a general warm-up, before another yoga session or if it's cold.

1. Toes

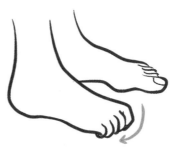

To wake up your toes, imitate a cat on your mat. Curl your toes in closer to your feet. Begin with the right, then move to the left. Then do both at the same time. Stand on tiptoes, first one foot then the other, and then both at the same time. Stretch to the sky, as high as you can!

Now lean back on your heels, first one then the other, then both at the same time. Do each of these exercises 10 times. As you do these movements, be very careful not to lose your balance.

2. Ankles

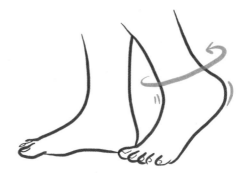

Start by making rotating movements with your ankles. Keep your toes on the floor, your heel up and the movement at ankle level. Rotate 10 times to the left, then 10 times to the right for each foot.

3. Knees

Bend your knees and place your hands on them. Make circles with your knees, 10 times one way and then 10 times the other, as if you were spinning a hoop around your knees.

Then stand on your right leg and lift your left leg up to the height of your pelvis, drawing circles in the air with your left foot one way and then the other, 10 times for each side. Then change legs. As you do these movements, be very careful not to lose your balance.

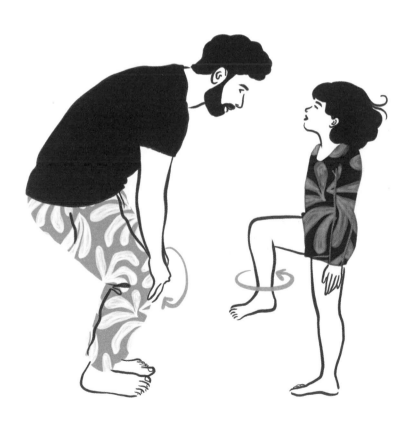

4. Pelvis

Put your hands on your hips with your feet apart. Move your pelvis to the right, then to the front, then to the left and then move it backwards. Do the movements in a fluid fashion as if you were spinning a hula hoop. Do them 10 times one way and then 10 times in the other direction.

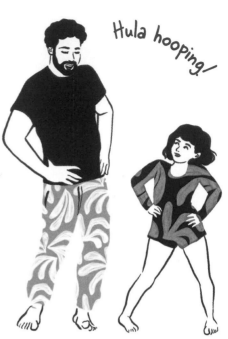

Hula hooping!

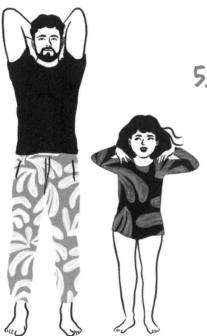

5. Shoulders

Place your hands on your shoulders and raise your elbows. Point them to the front, lower them so they are pointing downwards, then roll them out towards your back, narrowing your shoulder blades. Continue this circular movement, breathing in when your elbows are pointing backwards and breathing out when your elbows are facing forwards. Then change direction.

6. Elbows

Hold your arms out in front of you, parallel to the ground and palms to the sky. Bend your elbows and place your hands on your shoulders, then straighten your arms again. Repeat 10 times.

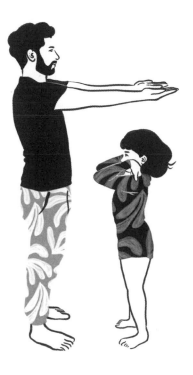

Imagine you have a scarf in each hand that you want to send shooting into the air with big wrist movements.

7. Wrists

Clasp your hands together with the fingers of each hand on the back of the other. Rotate your wrists first one way and then the other. One way will be easy and the other way a bit more difficult. Which way do you prefer?

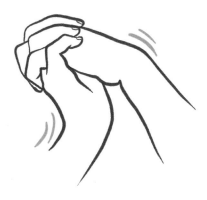

8. Fingers

Do you know the name for each of your fingers? Bend and stretch all your fingers at the same time, as if you were throwing a handful of glitter!

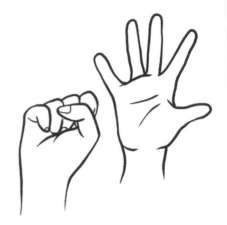

9. Neck

Tilt your head to the right, then the left, getting your ear close to your shoulder. Do this 10 times. Then nod your head up and down as if saying yes. Do that 10 times as well. Move your head to the left and right as if saying no. Do that 10 times. Now do all of those one after the other, making gentle, full rotations of the head clockwise. Breathe and relax your shoulders during these movements.

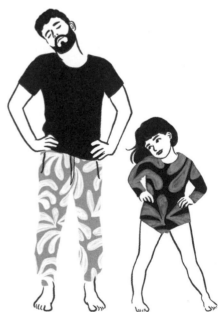

10. Upper back

Place your hands on your hips, arch your back and then curve it forwards. Use your shoulders to help you with the movement. Your shoulders move to the front when you curve forwards and move towards the back when you arch your back. Do not move your lower back!

With your hands still on your hips, move your upper back to the right, without moving the rest of the body. Then do the same thing to the left.

Then do these movements one after the other, moving your upper back in a circle, but keeping the rest of your body still. Rotate in one direction and then the other. Take your time and breathe carefully.

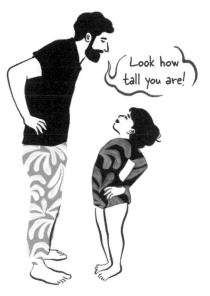

11. Lower back

Bend your knees slightly and curl over forwards to roll your spine forward. As you breathe out, bend your head over first, then your upper back and finally your lower back. Let your hands flop down in front of you. Relax your entire body forwards and breathe deeply. As you breathe in, unroll your back and slowly straighten up. Start with the lower back, then upper, shoulders and finally your head. Do this three times, taking the time to breathe deeply.

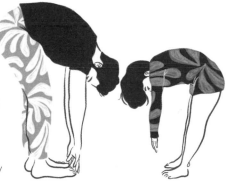

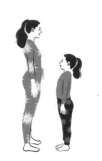

1. Mountain pose

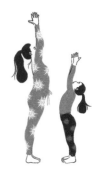

2. Catch the sun

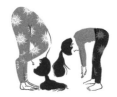

3. Forward fold

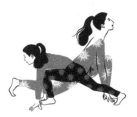

4. Warrior on one knee

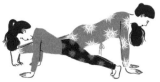

5. The plank

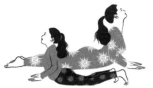

6. Little cobra

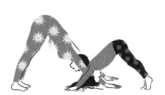

7. Downward-facing dog

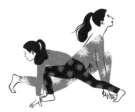

8. Warrior on one knee

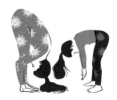

9. Forward fold

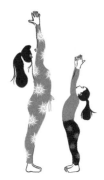

10. Catch the sun again

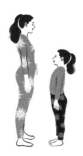

11. Mountain pose

Sun salutation

For all levels – perfect for beginners
For any time of day apart from the evening
Duration: 5 to 20 minutes

Yogis call this sequence 'surya namaskar'. It can be performed every morning by anyone, but should be avoided in the evening. It is dynamic and complete, as it uses all parts of the body. If you practise regularly, sun salutation can be performed as a warm-up for another sequence.

 This sequence of poses can be done standing face to face or side by side.

The poses can be done one by one, before you move on to doing them all in one long, continual, fluid movement, synchronising your breathing to the movements.

This sequence should be done twice, once starting on your right foot and again starting on your left foot.

When you know the sequence well, your child may want to perform it faster and faster, doing first one side and then the other. Yogis in India do it 108 times in a row. How many can you manage?

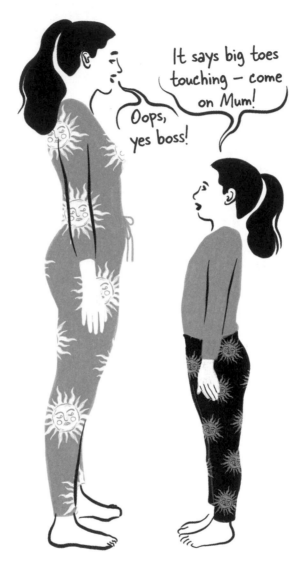

1. Mountain pose

Stand up straight, face to face, feet together with your big toes touching.

Make sure you stand tall, arms and legs straight, to create a really nice mountain, and take time to breathe in and out deeply.

2. Catch the sun

From the mountain pose, breathe in and place your hands together as if in prayer. Then, as you breathe out, lift your arms towards the sky as if catching the sun.

The stretch should be up towards the sky and not backwards, and you should keep your shoulders relaxed.

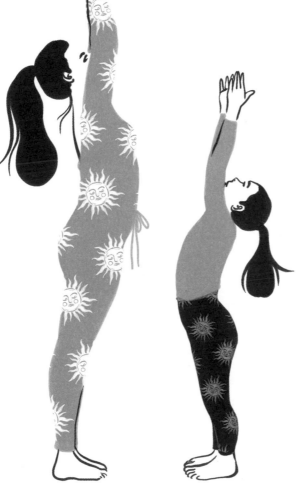

3. Forward fold

After you catch the sun, breathe in.

Then, as you breathe out, move your arms straight down to your feet, keeping your back straight, and touch the floor with your hands.

If your back hurts, bend your knees in order to put your hands on your ankles or shins, depending on what is comfortable for you.

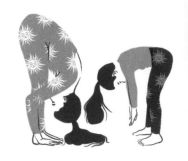

4. Warrior on one knee

After the forward fold pose, bend your knees, breathe in and put your hands on the floor in front of you. As you breathe out, move your right leg behind you, pressing your knee to the floor. Keeping your knee on the floor, straighten up your ribcage, look straight ahead of you and breathe in.

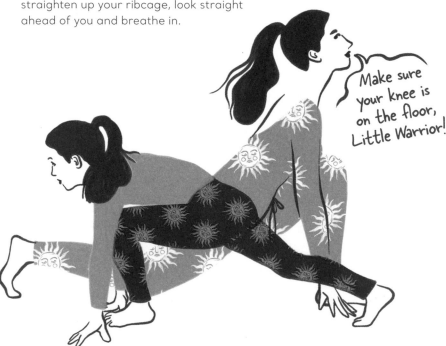

Make sure your knee is on the floor, Little Warrior!

5. The plank

Following the warrior on one knee pose, breathe out and move so your ribcage is parallel with the floor. Move your chin in, keep both arms straight, move both your feet to the back of the mat and straighten your legs. Keep your head straight at the top of your spine.

Your body will be in a straight line from the back of your neck to your feet. Breathing in and out deeply will help you stay in the pose.

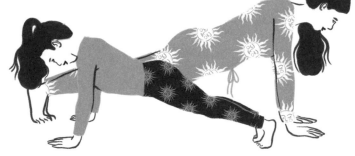

6. Little cobra

Breathe in and lie down on your front, with your arms and feet bent, and your hands below your shoulders. As you breathe out, lift your chest and your head while keeping your palms flat on the floor.

Breathe in deeply and, for the entire time you breathe out, imitate the hissing noise a snake makes, with your tongue behind your teeth.

Hold the pose while you have some fun.

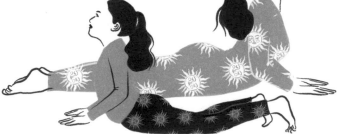

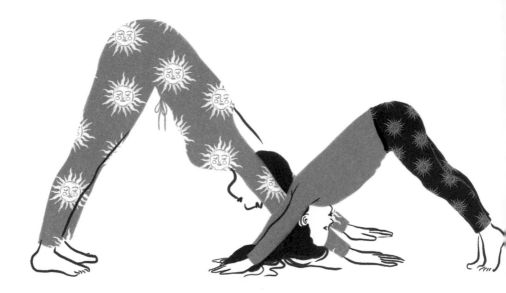

7. Downward-facing dog

After the little cobra pose, breathe out, and lower your head and ribcage to the floor. As you breathe in, push your hands so you lift your hips into the air to make an upside-down V shape with your body.

Your hands should be shoulder-width apart, and your fingers should be pointing forwards and spread out. Your knees should be the same width apart as your hips.

Push down hard with your hands, keeping your shoulders relaxed and your head tucked in. Look at your belly button.

Start with your toes on the floor. Then bend your right knee and stretch your left leg, lowering your left heel to the floor. Do the same on the other side and repeat this a few times. If you can, keep both heels on the floor.

You could start this one by getting into the pose and inviting your child to go underneath you. Then swap over. Help your child into the pose and take your turn going underneath. Can you pass underneath the downward-facing dog of your child?

8. Warrior on one knee

After the downward-facing dog pose, as you breathe out, place your right foot between your hands to resume the warrior on one knee pose (see 4, page 48).

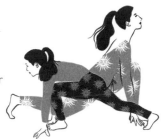

9. Forward fold

Bring your other foot forward between your hands at the front of the mat to get into the forward fold pose (see 3, page 48).

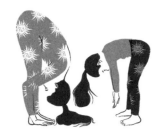

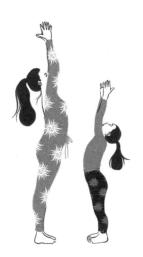

10. Catch the sun again

Following the forward fold, bend your knees and stand up, keeping your back and arms straight, to catch the sun (see 2, page 47).

11. Mountain pose

Return to this pose and repeat the sequence on the other side.

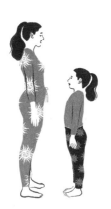

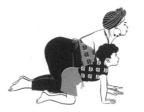
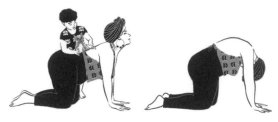

1. Cat on all fours

2. Cat with hollow back and rounded back

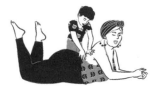
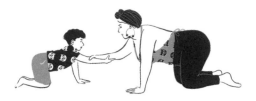

3. Massage cat

4. Cat stretching its paws forwards

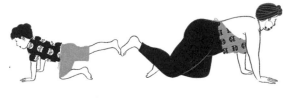

5. Cat stretching its paws backwards

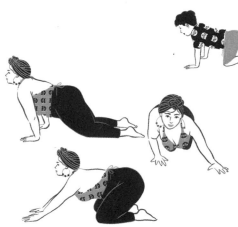
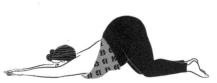

6. Cat movements

7. Heart-opening cat

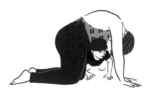
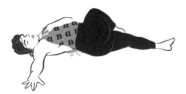

8. Cat bridge

9. Cat twist

10. Relaxation

The cat

For all ages
For all levels – perfect for beginners
For any time of day, ideal for relaxation
Duration: 10 to 15 minutes

For this sequence you are going to become a cat! Cats are very inspiring yogis!

This sequence is calm and relaxing, and can be done in the evening. It's an easy sequence, suitable for all.

1. Cat on all fours

Get on all fours. Place your hands on the floor shoulder-width apart with your fingers pointing forwards. Your knees should be the same width apart as your hips.

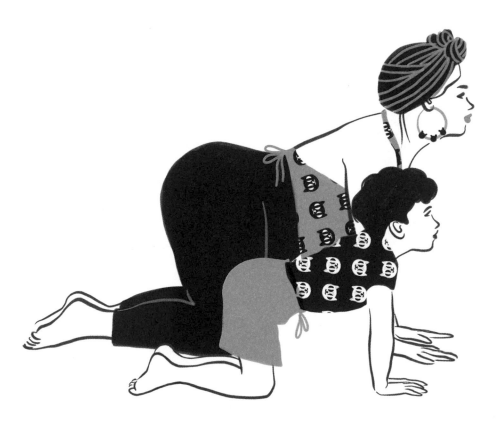

2. Cat with hollow back and rounded back

From the cat on all fours pose, breathe in, hollow your back and direct your buttocks towards the sky. Your head and neck should be stretched towards your back without straining them. Open out your ribcage and push your chin upwards and backwards, without relaxing the neck.

Then breathe out and round your back, direct your buttocks towards the floor and bring your chin towards your chest.

Continue moving between the two positions in a fluid, regular manner. Move the lower back first, the upper back second and the head last.

Start slowly and when you have a good rhythm established you can speed up the movements. Alternate between the two positions as quickly as you feel, always being careful to move the head last.

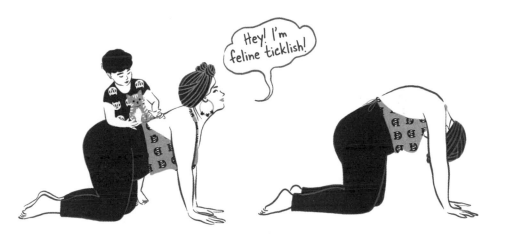

To start with you could show your child and ask them to put a soft toy on your back, to encourage them to take part and to see their toy go up and down with the rhythm of the movement. Then help your child to kneel next to you and do the pose. You can then put a soft toy on their back to see it go up and down with the movement. When your child can do it well, face each other and do the movements together.

3. Massage cat

Staying on all fours, with one hand and then the other, contract and relax your hands, in the way a cat kneads a cushion before sitting down or as if you want to carry off something you have caught.

Your child could do this on your back to give you a massage and then you could swap roles.

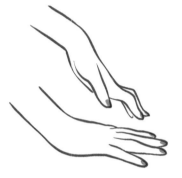

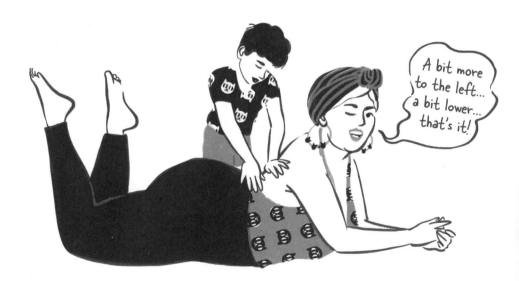

4. Paws forwards

Still on all fours, face each other, reach out an arm in front of you and hold your child's arm. You can make this a tug-of-war game if you like. Then swap arms.

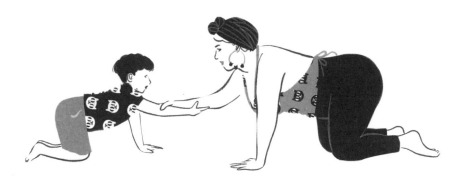

5. Paws backwards

Staying on all fours, turn away from each other. Like a cat who is just waking up, stretch out with a foot and place it on your child's foot. You can have fun taking turns pushing the other one's foot, which will bend your knee or straighten your leg. Then swap legs.

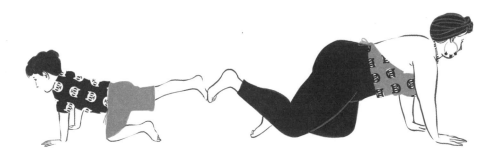

6. Cat movements

Staying on all fours with your hands on the floor and your knees in a comfortable position, bring your shoulders and ribcage towards the front as you look upwards.

Then move your weight to the right by bending your right arm and keeping your left arm straight.

Move your weight back, keeping both arms straight to make a good cat stretch. Move your hips back, but without sitting on your feet.

Then move to the left by bending your left arm and keeping your right arm straight.

Do this sequence on one side and then the other.

When your child is able to do all of the movements, you can perform this sequence in one continuous, fluid motion.

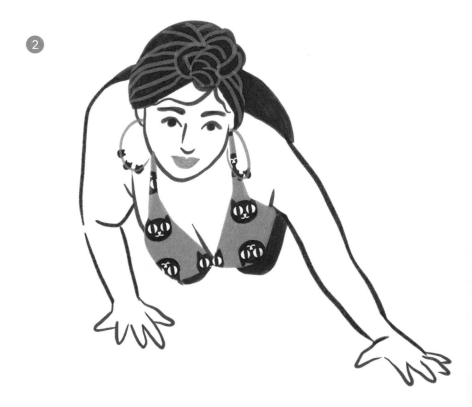

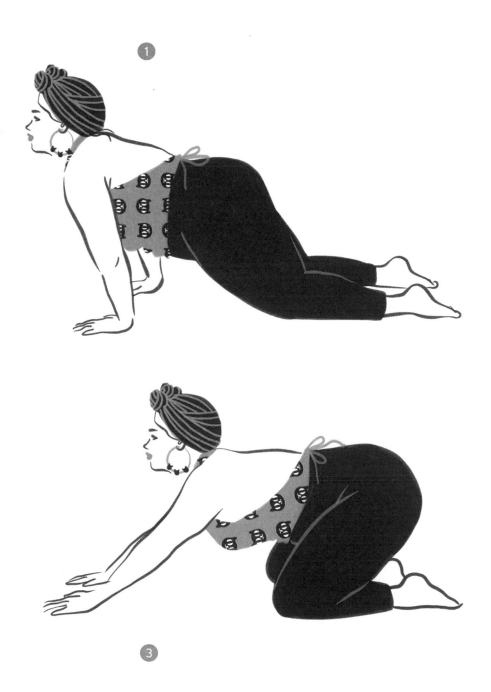

7. Heart-opening cat

Moving on from being on all fours, stretch your arms out in front of you as much as you can and lower your ribcage and chin gently down to the floor. Your pelvis remains up, pointing towards the sky, and your back is arched.

Face each other as you do this one and make sure your child has a good back posture.

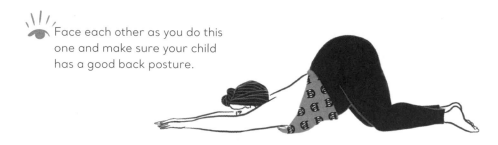

8. Cat bridge

Moving on to all fours, get yourself into a rounded back position, so your child can crawl underneath you.

Then it's your turn to crawl under them!

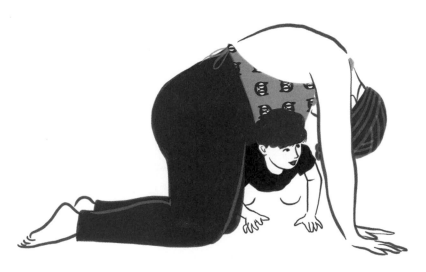

9. Cat twist

Lie on your back, arms out straight by your sides, in the shape of a cross.

Bring your right leg up to your chest and move the bent leg over to the left-hand side. Your left leg stays straight on the ground. Both shoulders should be flat on the floor and your head should be looking to the right.

Then change sides.

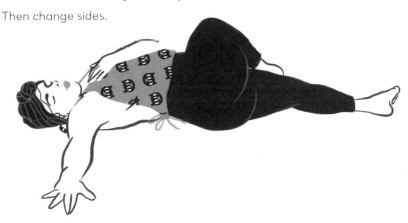

10. Relaxation

And now for some relaxation (for guided relaxation, see page 28).

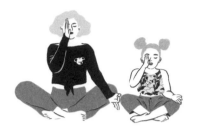

1. Koala breathing

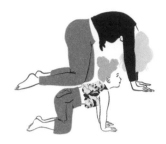

2. Koala copies a cat

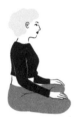

3. Koala bow

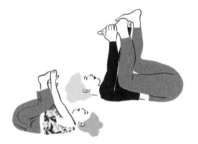

4. Baby koala

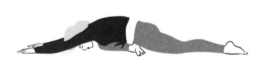

5. Koala stretch

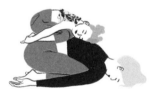

6. Young koala

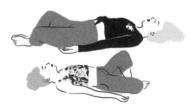

7. Koala resting like
a butterfly

The koala

For all levels – perfect for beginners
For any time of day, ideal for evening
Duration: 15 to 20 minutes

This session is good for bedtime preparation, with gentle poses and breathing that will help your child – and you – relax, stretch and restore.

It's night-time and we'll be going to bed soon!
Before we go off to dreamland we're going to
behave like a soft, cuddly koala bear.
As they sleep a lot, koalas don't move around
much and spend a long time in the same position.
We're going to do the same!

The koala takes its time to breathe calmly in a
special way, activating energy known as 'ida' from
the left-hand side of the body. Ida energy is calm
and relaxing.

1. Koala breathing

Sit in yogi pose. Place the back of your left hand on your
left knee, with your hand forming the 'gyan mudra', which
is made when the end of your thumb touches the tip of
your index finger.

Block your right nostril with your right thumb and, with
your fingers all pointing upwards, breathe in and then
out through your left nostril. Continue like this for at
least 10 breaths.

You can close your eyes or focus on the end of your nose.

You could make this a tender, cuddly moment by getting
your child to sit in the space between your legs.

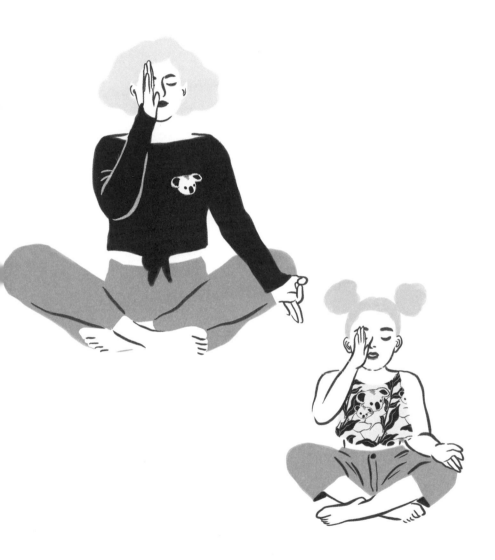

2. Koala copies a cat

Get down on all fours. Place your hands on the floor shoulder-width apart with your fingers pointing forwards. Your knees should be spaced the same width apart as your hips.

Breathe in, hollow your back and direct your buttocks towards the sky. Stretch your head and neck towards your back, but without straining them. Open out your ribcage and push your chin upwards and backwards, without relaxing your neck.

Without sitting on your feet, direct your buttocks towards the floor and bring your chin towards your chest.

Continue moving between the two positions in a fluid, regular manner. Move the lower back first, the upper back second and the head last.

Start slowly and when you have a good rhythm established you can speed up the movements. Alternate between the two positions as quickly as you can, always being careful to move the head last.

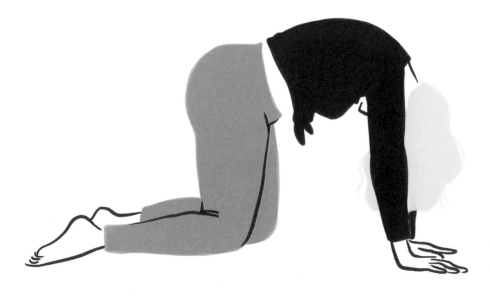

To start with, you could show your child and ask them to put a soft toy on your back, so they can watch it go up and down. Then, help your child to kneel next to you and do the pose. You can then put a soft toy on their back and watch it go up and down with their movements.

When your child can do it well, face each other and do the movements together. Before you change poses, encourage your child to go underneath you! Then swap places.

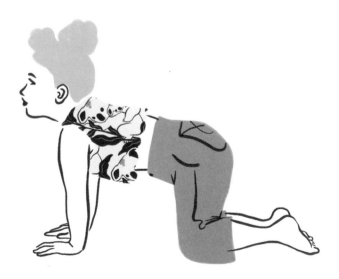

The koala night ritual lets you express your gratitude and appreciation from the heart, so your child can look back on their day, and tell you about what they learned and all the good things that happened to them. In order to take the time to really feel the gratitude, the koala takes a long moment in a reverential pose.

3. Koala bow

Sit in yogi pose.

Take the time while in yogi pose, face to face, to each express what you are grateful for.

In order to help, you could ask yourselves the following questions:

- Who do I feel grateful to?
- Who helped me today and who would I like to say thank you to?
- In what ways was I lucky?
- What were three good things that happened today?
- What did I see that was beautiful or positive today?
- Who would I like to thank?

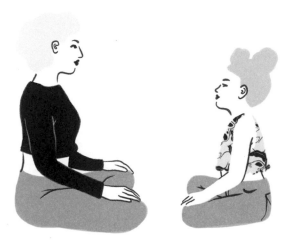

With your hands on the floor, gently tip your body forwards.

Take a long, deep breath and relax your body. Stay in this pose.

If this pose isn't comfortable and doesn't help you to relax, place your elbows on your knees and your hands together as if in prayer, and lower your head on to the top of your fingers.

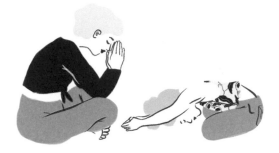

Before they go to bed, baby koalas make nothing but gentle movements. See if you can imitate a baby koala!

4. Baby koala

Lie on your back with your head on the ground. Grab the outside edges of your feet with your hands. Stay in this position for five deep inhalations and exhalations. Then, staying in the pose, ask your child to behave like a baby who's waking up and starting to move its feet, hands and body. Do the same yourself!

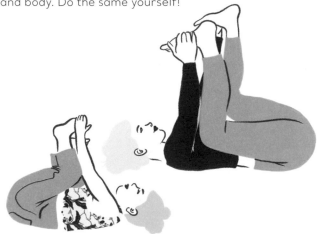

5. Koala stretch

To begin with, get into the downward-facing dog position (see page 50).

Bend your knees a little and bring your right foot up to the left. Put your right foot and right knee on the floor, and lower your hips. Your left leg is straight out behind you.

Bend over forwards and put your arms on the floor.

Stay like that for a few minutes and relax into the pose. Take long, deep breaths.

To get out of this position, take a deep breath, push down with your hands to bring your hips upwards and get back into the downward-facing dog position.

Bend your right knee a little, straighten your left leg and move your left heel so it touches the floor. Then do the same on the other side. Alternate one side and then the other. If you can, place both heels on the floor.

Then change legs and do this pose again.

If you can't touch the floor with your upper body and your head, place one or more cushions under your torso so you are still able to relax completely.

To continue your relaxation, get into young koala pose (see page 71).

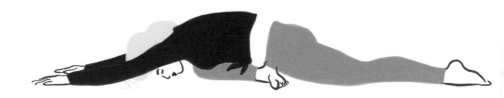

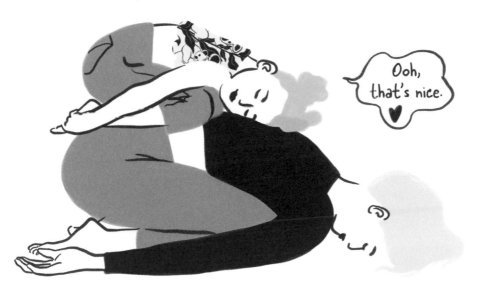

For little ones, and if your back is up to it, your child can do this while relaxing on your back.

Ooh, that's nice.

6. Young koala

Get on your knees and sit on your heels. Stretch your arms up and gently bring them down to the floor. Once your hands are on the floor, try to go as far forward as you can to really stretch out your back. Count to 10. Without getting up, bring your arms backwards along the length of your body to your feet and relax completely for a while in this pose.

To move on from this position, place your hands below your shoulders and gently, moving from the bottom of your spine first, rise up one vertebra at a time.

7. Koala resting like a butterfly

Lie on your back with your arms beside your body. Bend your knees and lower them to the floor on both sides. The soles of your feet should be together. Let yourself go, like a koala, and relax the whole of your body as you take long, deep breaths.

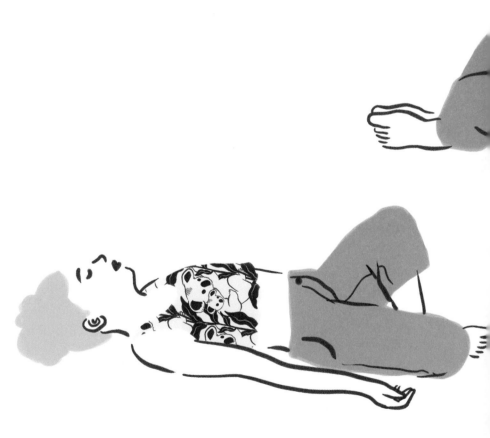

In order to be as relaxed as possible, you can put cushions under your knees to make this position more comfortable.

Your child can do this pose in their bed – they will be ready to sleep!

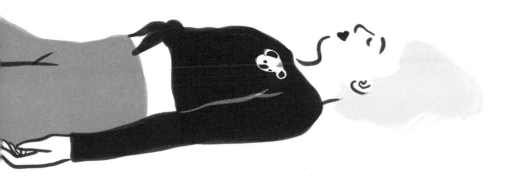

Stay in this position and relax (for guided relaxation, see page 28).

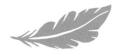

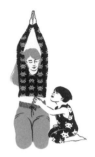

1. Switching on the strange magic machine

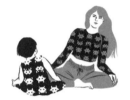

2. The big pump

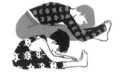

3. The clamp

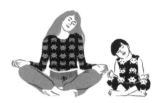

4. Little mixing programme

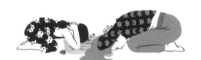

5. The big mix

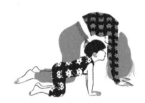

6. The cat

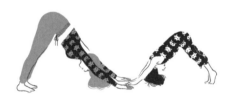

7. Downward-facing dog

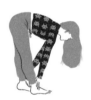

8. The elephant

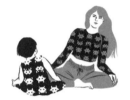

9. The strange magic machine slows down

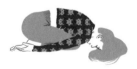

10. The machine stops

11. The song of the magic machine

12. Relaxation

The strange magic machine

For all ages
For all levels
For any time of day
Duration: 15 to 20 minutes

Yoga helps us develop our own internal resources. One of those is the ability to improve our health. This sequence will aid your digestion and ease stomach aches.

By using poses that encourage good digestive function, you can strengthen your resistance to illness.

This sequence is suitable for anyone, at any time of the day – even right before bed!

Take the time to be good to your belly while you have fun with this strange magic machine!

In order to get this strange magic machine going you need to start it with a little pump.

1. Switching on the strange magic machine

Get on your knees and sit down on your heels.

Put your hands above your head with your palms together.

Breathe in deeply to fully inflate your belly, then breathe out and bring your stomach in, as if you were a pump. This will massage your belly.

After 10 breath cycles sit down with your legs out in front of you, shaking them out and massaging them.

 Very young ones (four- to five-year-olds) can get into the pose with their hands on their hips instead of up in the air. The first time you do it you can show your child the movement and get them to put their hand on your belly, so they can feel it move – and switch on the little pump that starts the machine up. Then help your child into position and do it with them to make sure they do it correctly. You can then have a turn and place your hand on their belly as they activate the little pump. Finally, when they can do it well, sit face to face and do the movement together.

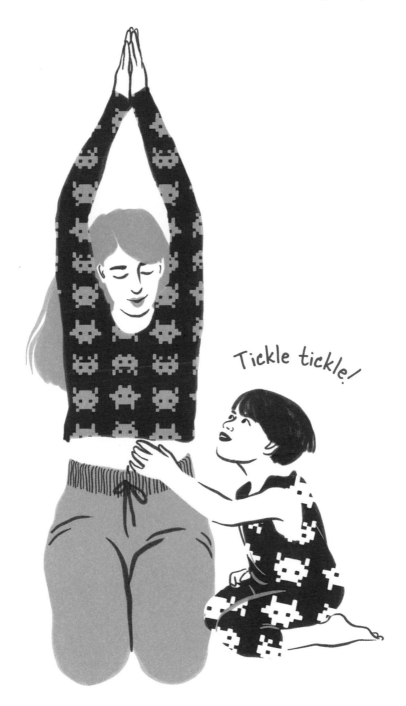

You have managed to switch on the strange magic machine and now the big pump will get going!

2. The big pump

As in the last pose, get on your knees and sit down on your heels.

Your fingers should be crossed in the Venus lock 'mudra' at the back of the neck.

To do the Venus lock 'mudra' cross all your fingers, but differently depending on whether you are a boy or a man or a girl or a woman. A man or boy should have their left little finger at the bottom and left thumb between the right thumb and index finger. A woman or girl should have the right little finger at the bottom and right thumb between the left index finger and thumb.

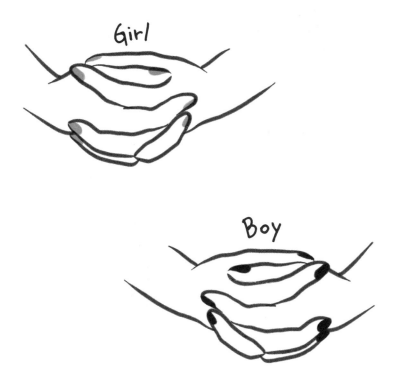

You have to do it to understand the subtle difference!

Breathe in and as you breathe out lean over forwards to put your forehead on the floor. Your buttocks should stay on your heels.

Breathe in and straighten up, then continue the movement.

When you have finished this pose you can sit up with your legs out in front of you, shaking them out and massaging them.

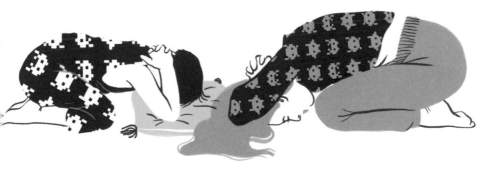

 Make the noise of a machine if you like!

As you lean over forwards, if you or your child are unable to reach the floor with your forehead you can put a cushion or two in front of you to rest on.

To change the programme on the strange magic machine we are going to use a big clamp!

3. The clamp

Sit down with your legs in front of you.

Stretch up from your back and, as you breathe in, lift both arms up to the sky. Then, as you exhale, fold over forwards gently and grasp your big toes, reaching round them with the index finger, middle finger and thumb of each hand.

Stay in this position and concentrate on your long, deep breathing.

Start with the lower back and continue to lower everything down further, keeping your spine long. Bend your head over last.

If you or your child are unable to grip your big toes, bend forwards and hold on to whatever you can (ankles, calves, knees). Keep a straight back and stretch your legs.

To start with, show this pose to your child. Then do it with them, making sure they keep their back straight. Then, you can do it together, in order to reprogramme the machine. Try it facing each other with your feet touching.

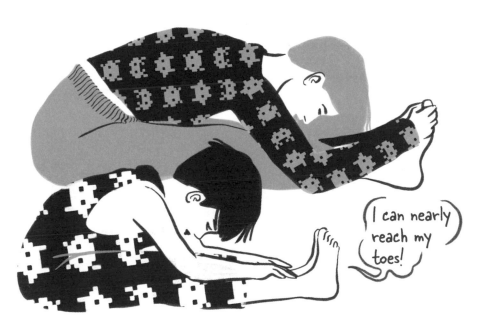

I can nearly reach my toes!

We've changed the programme on the strange magic machine and you can also use it for mixing. We're going to start with a little mixing programme on the head.

4. Little mixing programme

Sit in yogi pose with your shoulders relaxed.

To start mixing, gently rotate your head in a clockwise direction.

Synchronise your breath so you breathe in as your head moves round the back and breathe out as it goes to the front.

Then rotate your head in the other direction.

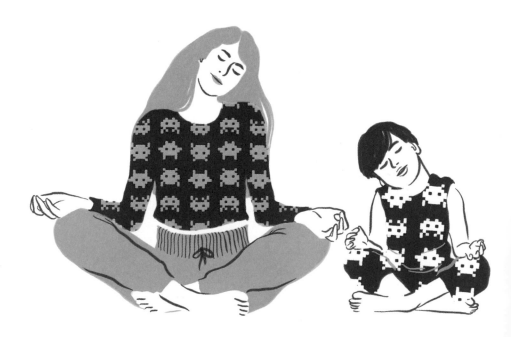

Now that we've done a little mixing cycle it's time to go bigger!

5. The big mix

Start in yogi pose.

Put your hands on your knees. Your shoulders should be relaxed.

Make big circles with your spine, breathing in as you move backwards and out as you move towards the front.

Your head should not move separately.

The top of your ribcage should stay open and don't let your head drop forwards.

To start with, do this with your child in front of you and do it with them to make sure they get into the right pose. When they can do it properly, face each other and mirror each other's movements. When you come face to face in the cycle, that could be the moment for a kiss!

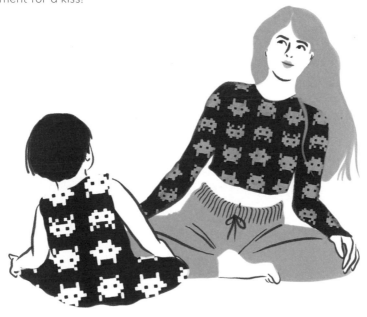

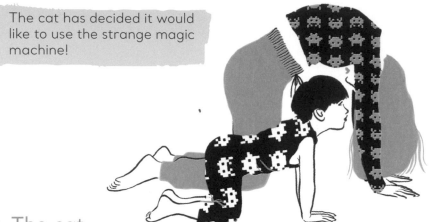

The cat has decided it would like to use the strange magic machine!

6. The cat

Get on all fours. Place your hands on the floor, shoulder-width apart and your fingers pointing forwards. Your knees should be spaced the same width apart as your hips.

Breathe in, hollow your back and direct your buttocks towards the sky. Your head and neck should be stretched towards your back without straining them. Open out your ribcage and push your chin upwards and backwards, without relaxing your neck.

Then breathe out and round your back, direct your buttocks towards the floor and bring your chin towards your chest. Move between the two poses in a fluid, regular manner. Move the lower back first, the upper back second and the head moving last.

Start slowly and when you have a good rhythm established you can speed up the movements. Alternate between the two positions as quickly as you feel, always being careful to move the head last.

To start with, you could show your child and ask them to put a soft toy on your back, to encourage them to take part and to see their toy go up and down with the rhythm of the movement. Then help your child to kneel next to you and do the pose. You can then put a soft toy on their back to see it go up and down with the movement.

When your child can do it well, face each other and do the movements together.

Now the dog is interested in the strange machine and has come over to see what's going on!

7. Downward-facing dog

Stand up. Bend over forwards and place your hands and feet flat on the floor. Take a big step back to make a large gap between your hands and feet. Push your hips upwards so you make an upside-down V shape with your body.

Your hands should be shoulder-width apart and your fingers should be spread out and pointing forwards. Your knees should be the same width apart as your hips.

Push down hard with your hands, shoulders relaxed, head tucked in, and look at your belly button.

Start with your toes on the floor. Then bend your right knee and stretch your left leg, lowering your left heel to the floor. Do the same on the other side and repeat this a few times. If you can, do it with both heels on the floor.

 You could start this one by getting into the pose and inviting your child to go underneath you. Then swap over. Help your child into the pose and take your turn going under. Can you pass underneath?

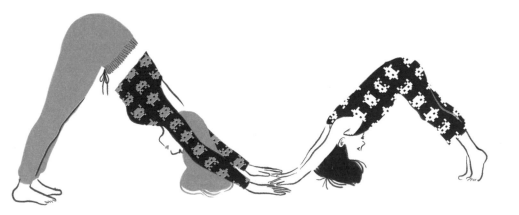

Surprise! An elephant has heard about this strange magic machine. Seeing as they have trouble digesting their meals, they want to use it, too.

8. The elephant

It's elephant time!

Stand up. Then bend over forwards and grab your ankles.

Without bending your knees, move around the room like this.

👁 Feel free to make a game of this by touching each other with your heads, but stay in elephant pose all the time.

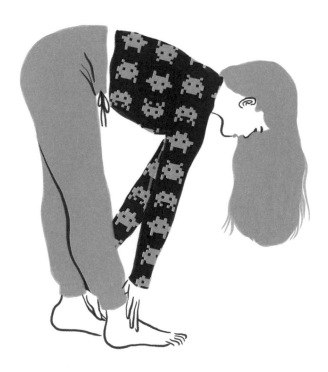

The strange magic machine doesn't switch off quickly, it slows down and breathes in a special way, using only energy from the left side of the body, known as 'ida'.

9. The strange magic machine slows down

Sit in yogi pose. Place the back of your left hand on your left knee with your hand forming the 'gyan mudra', which is made when the end of your thumb touches the tip of your index finger.

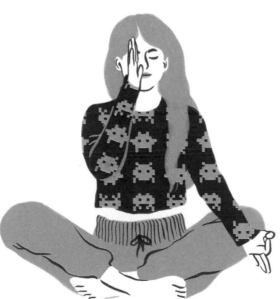

Block your right nostril with your right thumb, with your fingers all pointing upwards. Breathe in through your left nostril and breathe out through it as well. Continue like this for a dozen breaths.

You can close your eyes or focus on the end of your nose.

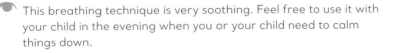

This breathing technique is very soothing. Feel free to use it with your child in the evening when you or your child need to calm things down.

10. The machine stops

Get on your knees and sit on your heels. Bend over forwards until your forehead touches the floor. Your arms should be next to your body, palms towards the sky.

This pose is commonly called child's pose. Stay in this position for a while for relaxation.

In order to get out of this pose, move your hands below your shoulders and uncurl your back slowly, starting with your lower back. Your head moves up last.

When you bend over, if you or your child can't reach the floor with your forehead you can place a cushion down and rest your head on that.

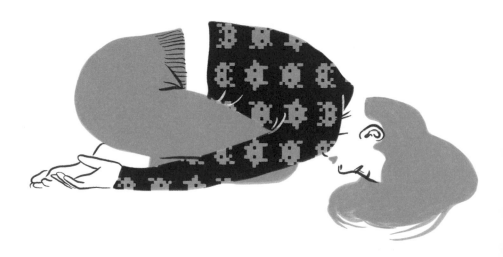

Now it has stopped, the strange magic machine starts singing.

11. The song of the strange magic machine

Sit in yogi pose. Bend your elbows so they are next to your ribs and your forearms make an angle of 45 degrees with the top of your body. Your hands should be parallel with the floor and your palms should face the sky. Your fingers should be together and your thumbs apart.

Stay in this position and chant the om sound three times (see page 21).

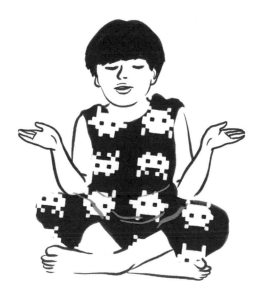

12. Relaxation

And now it's time for relaxation (for guided relaxation, see page 28).

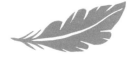

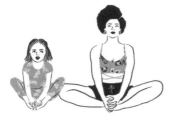

1. Little butterfly
feeding

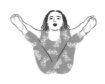

2. Little butterfly
gets bigger

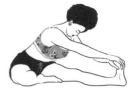

3. Butterfly flies with
just one wing

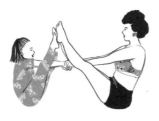

4. Watching butterflies
from a boat

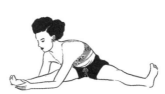

5. Steering the boat

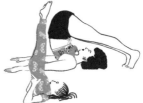

6. The candle

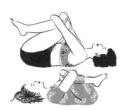

7. Rolling

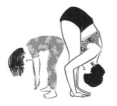

8. Forward folding
game

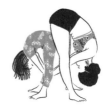

9. The upside-down
mirror game

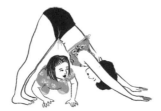

10. Downward-facing dog

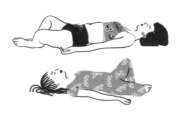

11. Butterfly resting

The butterfly

For all ages
For all levels
For any time of day
Duration: 15 to 20 minutes

Welcome to the world of butterflies. This sequence is based around leg stretching, and it can be done by anyone, at any time of day, including the evening.

1. Little butterfly feeding

Sit down with your back straight. Place the soles of your feet together and wrap your hands around your feet.

In this pose you are going to flap your little butterfly wings by moving your knees up and down vigorously.

This little butterfly needs to build their strength.

Stay in this position with your knees towards the floor and stretch upwards with your back, as if you were drinking water that's rolling off a leaf.

As you breathe out, bend forwards, keeping your back straight, and bring your body as close as you can to the floor, so the butterfly can drink the nectar from the flowers. Breathe in as you move back up and flap your wings again.

Repeat these stretches a few times to give your little butterfly plenty to eat and drink.

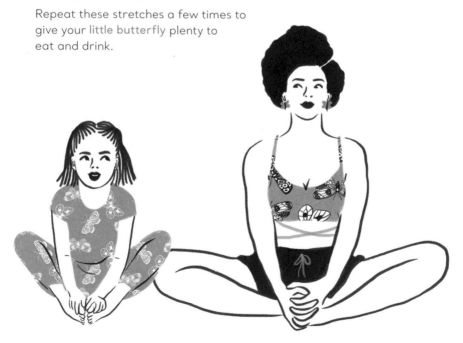

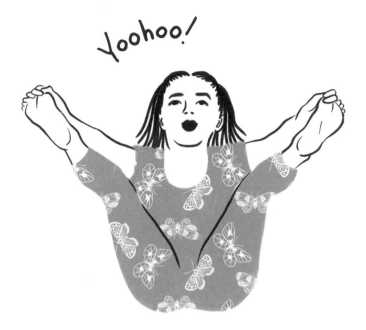

Now the little butterfly has learned to flap its wings and is full up, it grows bigger.

2. Little butterfly gets bigger

Staying seated, wrap your index fingers, middle fingers and thumbs around your big toes on each foot. As you breathe in, try to lift your legs upwards.

Stay in this position for a while, then bring your feet back to the floor.

Repeat a few times.

Some young butterflies find it funny to fly with only one wing. You can try it, too!

3. Butterfly flies with just one wing

Sit down with your left leg straight out on the floor and your right leg bent so your foot is resting at the top of your thigh. As you breathe in, lift both hands into the air. Then, as you breathe out, keeping your back straight, lower your torso, head and arms forwards.

Hold on to your foot or your shin, relaxing on to the leg.

Let yourself relax completely in this position with a long, deep breath.

Gently sit back upright, starting the upwards movement with your lower back and raising your head last.

Then change legs.

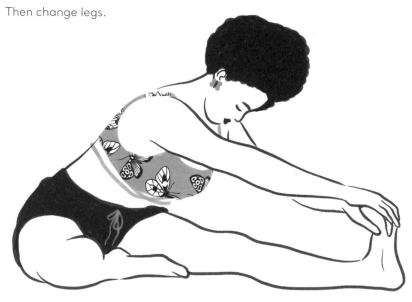

As you lower your body down, make sure that you keep your back straight and your head straight at the top of your spine. Go as far as you can without curling your back or lowering your head.

The butterflies we are watching have decided to fly over a pond. Let's get into a boat so we can see them!

4. Watching butterflies from a boat

Sit down facing each other. With your legs apart, put your feet together and hold each other's hands.

To row the boat, take turns to pull each other forwards, trying to reach as far as possible.

Continue this forwards and backwards movement and lean to the right. Come back to the centre and then lean to the left. Continue like this, but be careful not to fall in the water!

Still facing each other, get a bit closer and put your feet together, knees bent upwards, and hold hands.

Then, lift your feet up as high as you can inside your joined arms. Hold this position. Then try the same pose by lifting your feet up on the outside of your arms. Continue to raise your feet inside and outside, but – again – don't fall in the water!

 For the second part of the boat trip, start by just lifting one foot first, then the other, until you are well balanced enough to raise both at the same time.

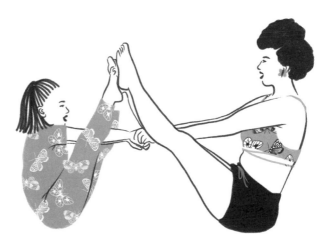

We are still watching the butterflies from our boat. To follow them, we need to go to the right, to the left, and sometimes we need to go straight ahead.

5. Steering the boat

Sit face to face with your legs apart and your toes pointing to the sky.

Take a deep breath and lift both your hands towards the sky. As you breathe out, lean forwards towards your right leg, keeping your back straight. Move your lower back first and your head last.

Hold your foot or, if you can't reach it, your calf or your knee. Stay in this position and take a long, deep breath.

To get out of this pose, take a deep breath and lift up slowly, starting with your lower back and lifting your head last.

Then change legs.

Come back to the centre.

From the same starting position, take a deep breath and lift both hands towards the sky. As you breathe out, lean over forwards, keeping your back straight. Watch each other as you go down. Move your lower back first and your head last.

Grasp each other's hands and, depending on how supple you are, you could hold on to each other's shoulders or even have a little kiss.

To get out of this position, take a deep breath and lift up slowly, starting with the lower back and moving your head last.

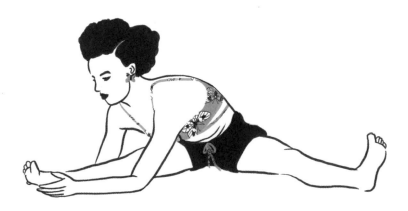

The butterflies have flown away. We'll go back to the shore to do some exercise while we wait for them to come back!

6. The candle

Lie on your back with your arms beside your body, palms down.

Raise your legs so they are at an angle of 90 degrees to the floor. Lift your pelvis up to get into candle pose. Put your hands on your lower back, elbows on the floor.

Take long, deep breaths to help you stay in this position.

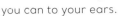

With very young children, or those who aren't used to this, help them the first time by lifting their legs and holding them as straight as possible. Also help them to get out of this position by carefully lowering them back to the floor. Women shouldn't do this pose if they are pregnant or at the start of their menstrual cycle.

Next, gently lower your straight legs to behind your head. Stay in this position and, if you can, put your toes on the floor. Breathe.

Then stay in this pose and spread your legs. Breathe.

Bring your legs back together and bend your knees in order to get them as close as you can to your ears.

To get out of this position, keep your knees bent and gently bring your legs back in front of you. Stay lying down for a little while.

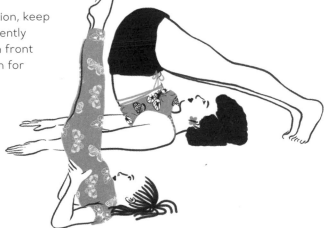

97

To give us a massage after all that effort we're going to roll around in the grass!

7. Rolling

Lie on your back and hold your knees to your chest.

Rock backwards and forwards.

On the last roll, make a bigger movement to rock you up into sitting position or, if you can, standing up.

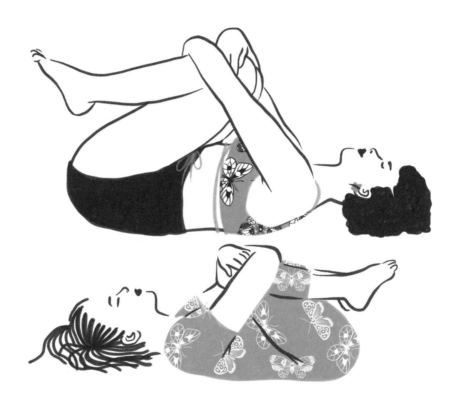

The butterflies are back! They are flapping around us and it looks like they want to play! Let's make some big movements to play with them.

8. Forward folding game

Stand up, back to back, with your feet together and shoulders relaxed.

Breathe in and raise your arms upwards. As you breathe out, lower your arms, straight towards your feet, keeping your back straight.

When you are down, relax your back and your arms, and place your hands on the floor.

If your back feels tight, bend your knees so you can put your hands on your ankles or shins, whatever is comfortable.

Stay in this pose, taking long, deep breaths.

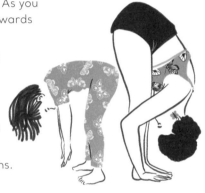

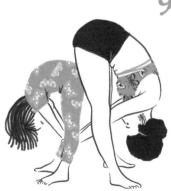

9. The upside-down mirror game

Staying in the forward fold pose, spread your legs in order to make a tunnel and hold each other's hands. Take turns to gently pull each other forwards to help stretch the backs of your legs.

Stay in this pose, taking long, deep breaths.

10. Downward-facing dog

From the upside-down mirror pose, let go of each other's hands and put your hands in front of you to get into downward-facing dog pose.

Bend over forwards and place your hands and feet flat on the floor, your hips in the air, so you make an upside-down V shape with your body.

Your hands should be shoulder-width apart and your fingers should be pointing forwards with your fingers spread out. Your knees should be the same width apart as your hips.

Push down hard with your hands, shoulders relaxed, head tucked in, and look at your belly button.

Start with your toes on the floor. Then bend your right knee and stretch the left leg, lowering your left heel to the floor. Do the same on the other side and repeat this a few times. If you can, have both heels on the floor.

You could start this one by getting into the pose and inviting your child to go underneath you. Then swap over, help your child into the pose and it's your turn to go under – what happens?

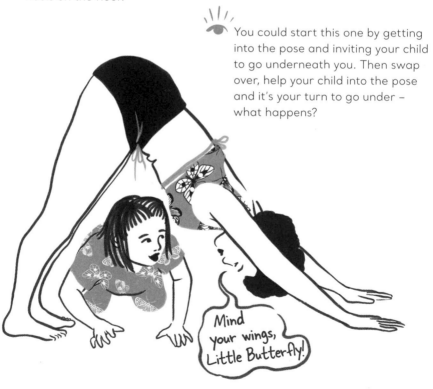

Mind your wings, Little Butterfly!

Now the butterflies need a rest.

11. Butterfly resting

Lie on your back with your arms beside your body. Bend your knees and lower them to the floor. Put the soles of your feet together. Let yourself unwind into the restful state of a butterfly by relaxing every part of your body and taking long, deep breaths.

Stay in this position and relax (for guided relaxation, see page 28.)

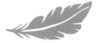

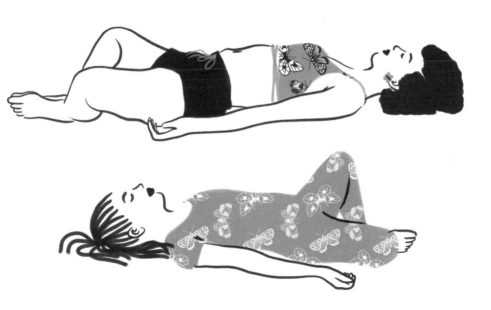

In order to be as relaxed as possible, you can put cushions under your knees to make this position more comfortable.

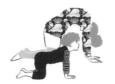 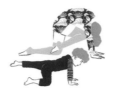 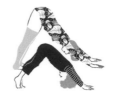

1. Up you get cat – time to wake up!

2. The backwards-kicking cow

3. The dog comes too

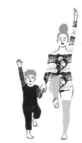 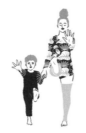 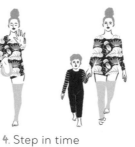 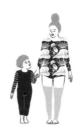

4. Step in time

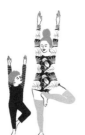 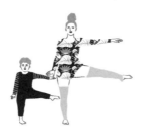 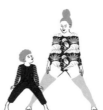 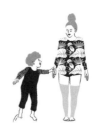

5. Sidestep

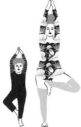 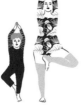 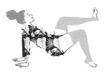 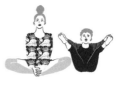

7. The bridge

8. The spider

9. Butterflies

6. The tree

   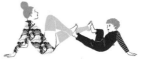

11. Boat trip on the pond

12. Learning to row

13. Back on bikes

10. Frogs

14. Garden rollers

15. Relaxation

A walk by
the pond

For all ages
For all levels
For any time of day, apart from the evening
Duration: 25 to 30 minutes

Today we are going for a family walk to the pond. There should be lots of creatures to meet and a few surprises! This sequence awakens different parts of our bodies. It burns off some excess energy or gives us an energy boost for the day.

It's an ideal sequence for the morning and suitable for the afternoon too.

On our way we come across a cat lying in the sun. The cat decides to join us!

1. Up you get cat – time to wake up!

Get on all fours. Place your hands on the floor shoulder-width apart and with your fingers pointing forwards. Your knees should be spaced the same width apart as your hips.

Inhale and tilt your hips towards the sky and hollowing the back. Your head and neck should be stretched towards your back without straining them. Open out your ribcage and push your chin upwards and backwards.

Then breathe out and hollow your back, moving your hips upwards and bringing your chin towards your chest.

Continue moving between the two poses in a fluid, regular manner. Then exhale and make the back round, moving your hips to the ground and bringing your chin to your chest.

Start slowly and when you have a good rhythm established you can speed up the movements. Alternate between the two positions as quickly as you can, always being careful to move the head last.

To start with, you could show your child and ask them to put a soft toy on your back, to encourage them to take part and to see their toy go up and down with the rhythm of the movement. Then get your child to kneel next to you and help them to do the pose. You can then put a soft toy on their back to see it go up and down.

When your child can do it well, face each other and do the movements together.

Before you move on, you could ask your child to be a cat and walk beneath you while you round your back. Then change places.

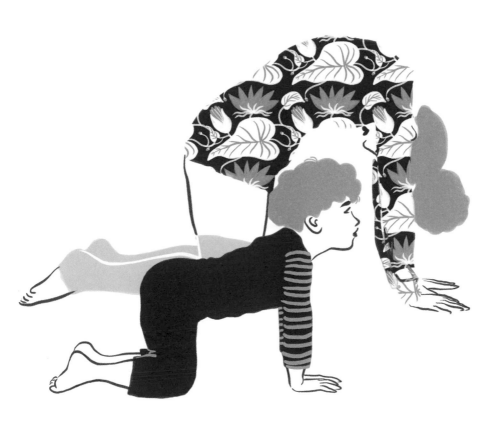

While crossing the meadow we come across a nice cow, who is waking itself up with some backwards kicks.

2. The backwards-kicking cow

Get on all fours. Place your hands on the floor shoulder-width apart and with your fingers pointing forwards. Your knees should be spaced the same width apart as your hips.

Breathe in and lift your head up, at the same time stretching out your right leg behind you.

Then, as you breathe out, bring your right knee up to your chest while you drop your head in the direction of your knee.

Continue like this and then change legs.

As you breathe out, you could have fun by mooing like a cow. You can face each other and start a cow conversation together.

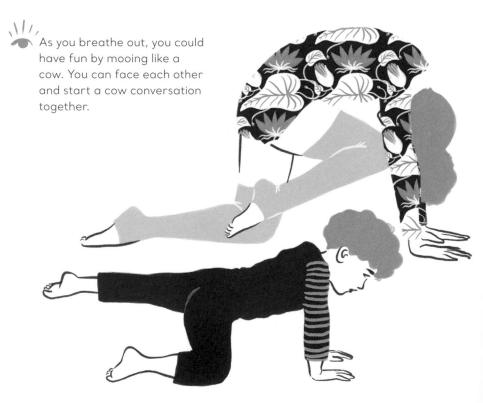

We've just realised that our dog has followed us. In order to persuade us to let him come on the walk with us, he greets us with the downward-facing dog pose.

3. The dog comes too

Get on all fours. Push hard with your hands and your feet so you lift your hips into the air to make an upside-down V shape with your body.

Your hands should be shoulder-width apart and your fingers should be spread out and pointing forwards.

Your knees should be the same width apart as your hips. Push down hard with your hands, shoulders relaxed, head tucked in, looking at your belly button.

Start with your toes on the floor. Then bend your right knee a bit and stretch your left leg, lowering your left heel to the floor. Do the same on the other side and repeat this a few times. If you can, have both heels on the floor.

To start with, get into the pose and invite your child to go underneath you. Then swap over. When it's your turn to go under, can you fit?

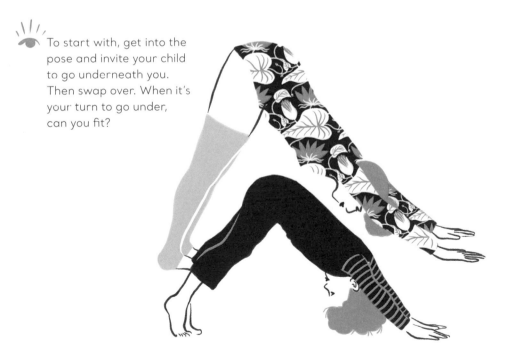

We decide to turn our walk into a game and get into step.

4. Step in time

Stand side by side, holding hands.

As you breathe in, lift your right knee to your chest and your left hand to the sky.

Breathe out in two parts. First straighten your right leg to be horizontal and lower your left arm to be parallel to it. Then drop your right foot to the floor as you bring down your left arm and move your left foot forward so it's next to your right foot. Continue in this way and then change sides.

Remember to concentrate!

 Your child should do the same movement with the opposite arm and leg to you.

Synchronise your movements so you have the same rhythm and then go faster without getting muddled up.

You can accompany your movements with the mantra SA TA NA MA:

SA as you lift the leg and arm;

TA when arm and leg are horizontal;

NA when the foot touches the floor and the arm comes down; and

MA as the foot that was behind moves next to the forward foot and both arms are next to your body.

This mantra represents the cycle of creation, the cycle of life.

SA is the beginning, the infinite, the cosmos.

TA is life, existence.

NA is death, change, transformation.

MA is rebirth.

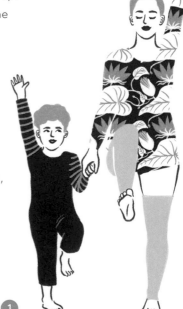

1

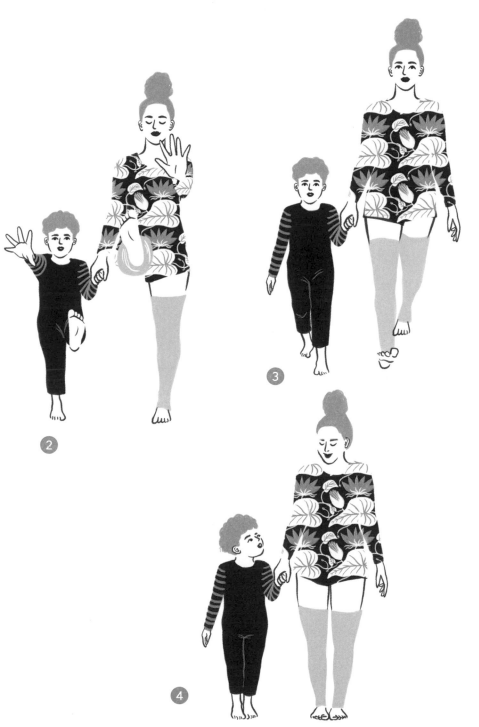

We are going to continue our stroll with another unusual style of walking!

5. Sidestep

Stand next to each other.

At the same time, lift your left knee to hip level and both arms towards the sky.

Straighten your left arm and leg horizontally out to the left.

Then bring your arm down and put your left foot down on the floor, with your legs apart.

Jump together as you lift your arms.

Continue to walk like this and then change sides.

 Your child should do the same movement with the same leg as you.

Synchronise your movements and move forwards with the same rhythm. Then change sides.

Remember to concentrate!

You can accompany your movement with the mantra SA TA NA MA:

SA as you lift your leg and arms;

TA as you move your leg to the side;

NA as you put your foot back down; and

MA as you jump.

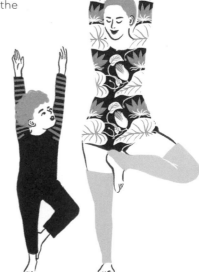

1

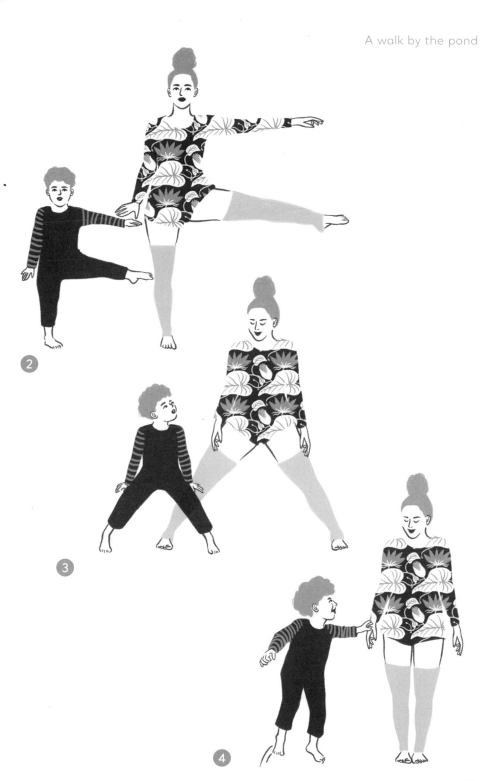

After this energetic walking we stop in the forest to rest and look at the trees. There are big ones, very big ones and small ones. Some have broad trunks and others have narrow trunks. They all have different branches and leaves, but each one seems to have its place and its role in the forest. Now you're going to become a tree!

6. The tree

Stand next to each other with your weight on your right foot and your left foot on the calf or thigh of your right leg.

Your right leg should be straight, stable and anchored to the floor, like the trunk of a tree. Your left foot should be carefully planted on your right leg – it is a branch of the tree.

Lift both hands towards the sky as if they were two more branches.

Stay balanced in this position and breathe deeply.

If you are comfortable like this, you can move your arms as if they are branches moving in the wind.

Then put your left foot back on the floor and change sides.

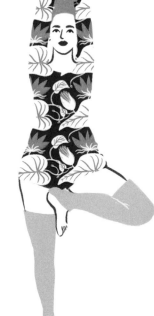

Don't put your foot on the opposite knee, because that's a joint and if you press too hard it could be painful! To have a bit of fun, you can get into tree pose and ask your child to test your stability by tickling you. Remind them you get to swap roles afterwards though!

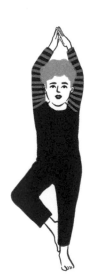

After that little rest, we carry on our way and cross a nice bridge.

7. The bridge

Your body is going to make a bridge.

Sit down, legs out on the floor. Bend your knees with your feet flat on the floor, hip-width apart.

Place your arms behind your body, palms flat on the floor, fingers pointing in the direction of your feet. Lift your hips to make a nice, straight bridge.

Your chin should be in a straight line with your chest in order to keep your head in the same line as your body.

Use your breathing to help you hold the pose.

To start with, help your child to get into position. You can make stuffed toys or cars go under the bridge.

Then you can get into position and your child can make sure that the bridge is nice and straight, and have fun going under it themselves!

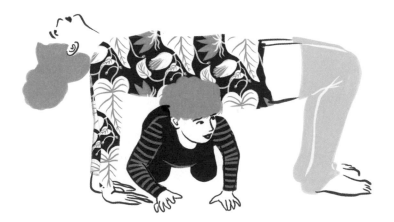

Under the bridge a spider beckons us over and asks us to follow it. It will lead us to the pond.

8. The spider

From the bridge pose, lower your hips, but don't let them touch the floor. Walk around like this and try to touch each other with your big toes. Then come back to your mat.

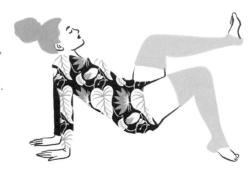

At last we've reached the side of the pond, where we can see the lovely, whirling butterflies.

9. Butterflies

Sit down with your back straight. Put the soles of your feet together and hold your feet with your hands.

In this pose, flap your little butterfly wings energetically by moving your knees up and down.

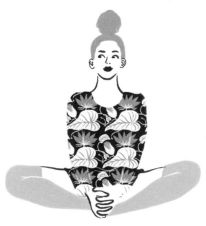

This little butterfly needs plenty of sustenance.

Keeping the same position, with your knees down, stretch your spine upwards as if you were drinking some water running off a leaf.

As you breathe out, bend over forwards and move your body as low as you can so the butterfly can drink nectar from the flowers.

Breathe in as you lift up and flap your wings again.

Repeat these stretches a few times so the little butterfly has enough to eat and drink.

Now the little butterfly has learned to flap its wings and is full, it becomes a big butterfly.

Stay seated, wrap your index fingers, middle fingers and thumbs around the big toes on each foot and try to stretch your legs up to the sky.

Stay in this position for a while, then bring your feet back to the floor.

Repeat a few times.

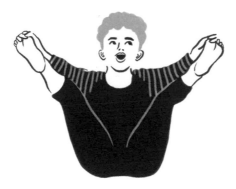

On the shore of the pond we come across a family of funny frogs. Let's copy their movements.

10. Frogs

Stand facing each other, with your heels together. Crouch down on your toes, keeping your heels together. Put your hands between your legs, with your fingers on the floor.

Keep your head up, look at each other.

Breathe in and lift your hips towards the sky and lower your head. Look at your knees and keep your heels up.

Breathe out and come back to your starting position, crouching down.

Do this movement a few times.

Once you have done this movement a few times, you can have fun by doing some forward jumps in order to leap into the pond.

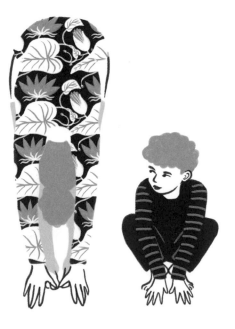

Now let's take a boat trip on
the pond!

11. Boat trip on the pond

Climb aboard the boat and sit facing each other.

With your legs flat on the floor, put your feet together and hold each
other's hands.

To row the boat, take turns to pull each other forward, trying to reach
as far as possible.

Continue this forwards and backwards movement and lean to the
right. Come back to the centre and then lean to the left. Continue like
this, but be careful not to fall in the water!

Still facing each other, get a bit closer and put your feet together, knees
bent upwards, and hold hands.

Then lift your feet up together, inside your joined arms. Hold this
position and breathe. Then try the same position, lifting your feet up on
the outside of your arms. Continue to raise your feet inside and outside,
but – again – don't fall in the water!

For the second part of the boat trip, start by lifting
one foot first, then the other, until you are well
balanced enough to raise both at the same time.

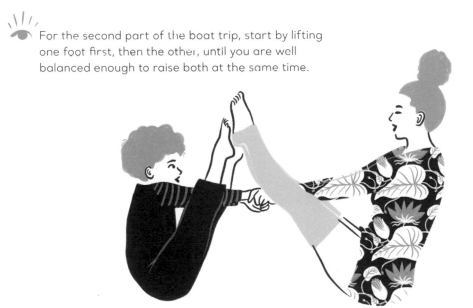

After the boat, let's try a different type of craft and learn another way of rowing!

12. Learning to row

Sit down with your legs apart, straight out in front of you, you behind your child.

Lean forwards together, arms held horizontally as you breathe in. Then, as you exhale, clench your hands into fists and bring them back to your armpits and lean back, taking care not to arch your back.

Continue this, moving rhythmically forwards and backwards together.

Tense your abs to avoid arching your back.

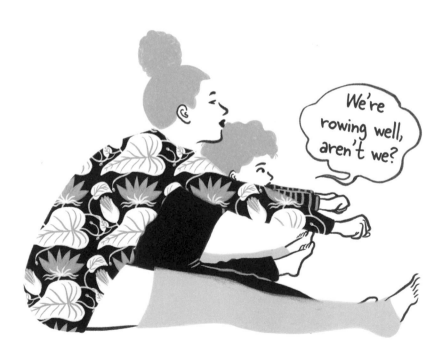

It is time to go home. Let's get on our bikes for the journey back!

13. Back on bikes

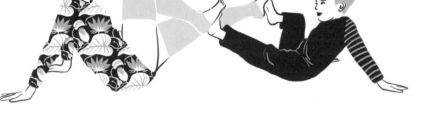

Sit facing each other. Put your hands on the floor behind you with your arms straight. Put the soles of your feet together, push your feet one by one and pedal!

Wheely good, isn't it?

We are back home after a lovely walk! Let's have some fun doing some rolling in the garden.

14 Garden rollers

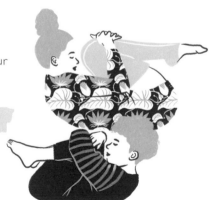

Lying on your back, hold your knees to your chest, and roll forwards and backwards.

We had a great walk and are getting ready for a well-earned relaxation session!

15. Relaxation

And now, time for relaxation (for guided relaxation, see page 28).

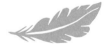

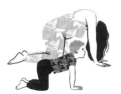 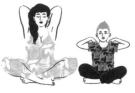

1. The cat and the fairy

2. Uncurling the fairy's wings

3. Small fairy wing rotations

4. Big fairy wing rotations

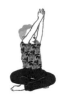 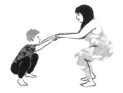 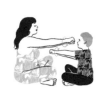 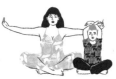

5. Dancing fairy rotations

6. The fairy's yogi squats

7. Fairy twist

8. Fairy wings up and down

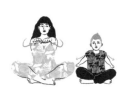 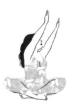 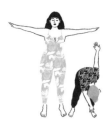 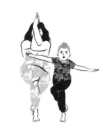

9. Fairy wings front to back

10. Fairy wings to the side

11. Small fairy arm rotations

12. Big fairy parade

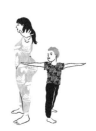 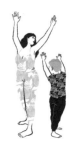 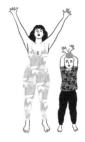

13. Fairy whirl

14. Standing fairy spreads wing to the side

15. Fairy bow

16. A visit from his friend the eagle

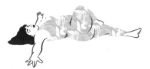

17. Lying down fairy twist

18. Relaxation

The fairy

For all ages
For all levels
For any time of day, apart from the evening
Duration: 25 to 30 minutess

This session helps strengthen muscles in the arms and the spine, as well as aiding mobility, circulation and digestion. It is recommended for morning or afternoon.

Today we are going to follow a fairy into her world! She's very lively, and looks at everything that's going on around her as she flits from place to place to visit her friends and everyone who needs her!
To start with, the fairy and her cat do some stretches.

1. The cat and the fairy

Get on all fours. Place your hands on the floor shoulder-width apart with your fingers pointing forwards. Your knees should be the same width apart as your hips.

Breathe in, hollow your back and push your bottom towards the sky. Your head and neck should be stretched towards your back without straining them. Open out your ribcage and push your chin upwards and backwards, without relaxing your neck.

Then breathe out and round your back, direct your bottom towards the floor and bring your chin towards your chest. Continue moving between the two poses in a fluid, regular manner. Move the lower back first, the upper back second and the head last.

Start slowly and when you have a good rhythm established you can speed up the movements. Alternate between the two positions as quickly as you feel, always being careful to move the head last.

To start with, you could show your child and ask them to put a soft toy on your back to encourage them to take part and to see their toy go up and down with the rhythm of the movement.

Then, help your child kneel next to you and to get into position. You can then put a soft toy on their back to see it go up and down with the movement.

When your child can do it well, face each other and do the movements together.

Before you move on, ask your child to crawl underneath you! Then swap over.

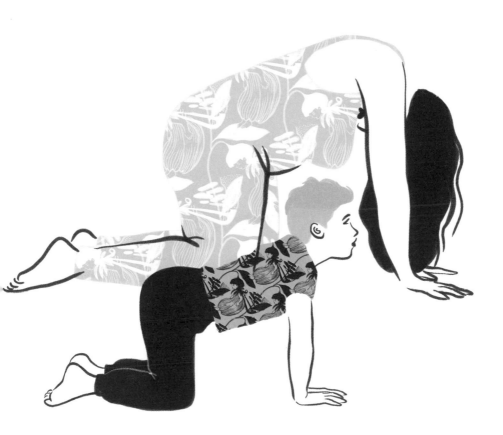

In order to be as fast and lively as the fairy, we're going to do some special arm exercises.

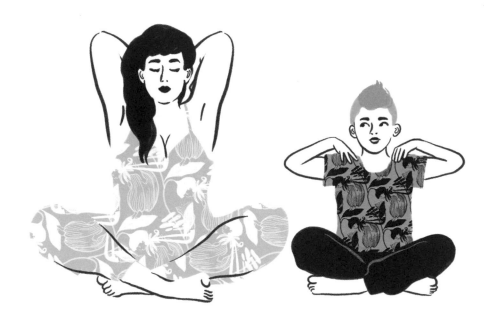

2. Uncurling the fairy's wings

Sit in yogi pose, facing each other or side by side.

Put your hands on your shoulders, lift your elbows, then move them in front of you and down, bringing them together before moving them behind you so your shoulder blades move towards each other. Continue this circular movement, breathing in when your elbows are behind you and breathing out when your elbows are in front of you.

Then change direction.

3. Small fairy wing rotations

Staying in the same pose as before, breathe in and turn your upper body to the left, making sure your head and arms move too. As you breathe out, do the same thing, but to the right. Continue to synchronise the movement with your breathing.

 If you are facing each other, you can wink or smile as you come back to the centre.

When your child is older, ask them to close their eyes and to focus their attention on the point between their eyebrows.

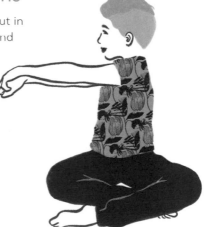

4. Big fairy wing rotations

Sitting in yogi pose, hold your arms out in front of you horizontally, with one hand on top of the other.

As you breathe in, turn your upper body to the left by moving your outstretched arms to the left. Your head should follow the movement.

As you breathe out, do the same movement to the right.

Continue to synchronise the movement with your breathing.

5. Dancing fairy rotations

Sitting in yogi pose, stretch your arms to the sky,
palms together.

As you breathe in, rotate your body to the left.

Your hands and head should follow the body's movement.

As you breathe out, do the same movement to the right.

Continue to synchronise the movement with
your breathing.

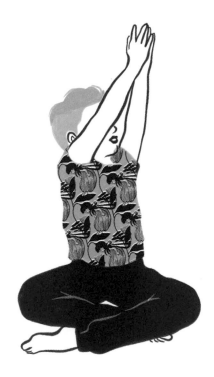

The fairy catches her breath in squatting position.

6. The fairy's yogi squats

Crouch down facing each other and hold each other's hands.

Help each other find your balance and, if possible, keep your heels on the floor.

This exercise is often easier for children than it is for parents!

Move your feet and find the right distance apart for your legs. Some people find yogi squats easy with their feet together, others don't. Do whatever you can manage.

When you have found a comfortable position, check how stable it is by letting go of your child's hands. If you fall over, try again!

Stay and breathe in this position.

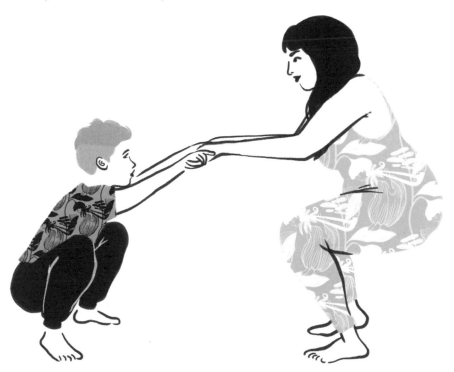

The fairy spins one way and then the other. She does twisting, stretching exercises.

7. Fairy twist

Sit back to back with your legs out in front of you.

Bend your right knee and place your right foot on the floor on the outside of your left leg. Hold your right knee with your hands, keeping your back and head straight. The toes of your left leg should be pointing upwards.

Stay and breathe in this position.

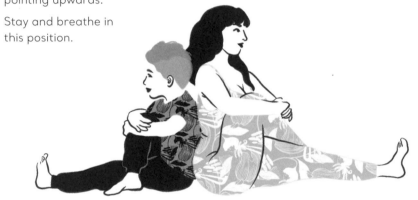

Then turn your upper body to the right. Put your left elbow behind your right knee, pointing the fingers of your left hand to the sky. Put your right hand on the floor behind your hip and look backwards – you can see each other!

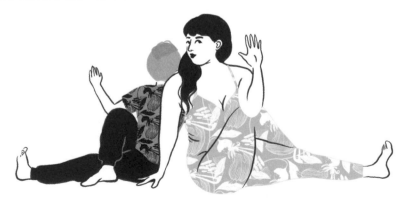

As you breathe in, turn your body to the right. Your arms and head should follow the movement. Stay and breathe in this position.

If you can, from this position, put your left hand under your right knee. Still keeping your back straight, move your right arm behind your back and hold your left hand. Your head should be looking backwards, to the right.

Stay and breathe in this position.

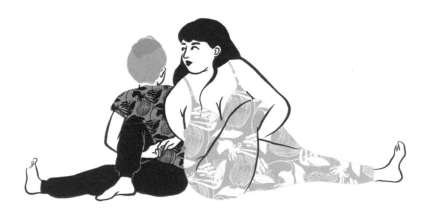

Release slowly and put both legs out in front of you again.

Then do the whole thing on the other side.

That's it – the fairy is ready to spread her wings in all directions!

8. Fairy wings up and down

Sitting in yogi pose, hold your arms out horizontally to the side with your hands perpendicular to your arms, fingers pointing to the sky, palms towards you. Breathe in.

As you breathe out, cross your arms behind your head.

Repeat this movement at least 10 times in time with your breath.

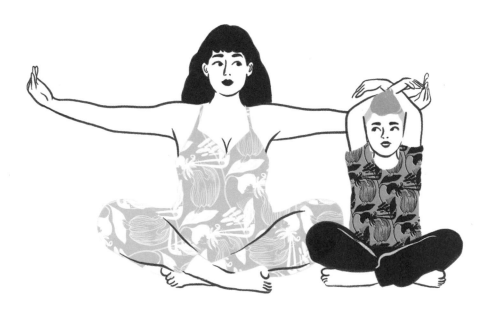

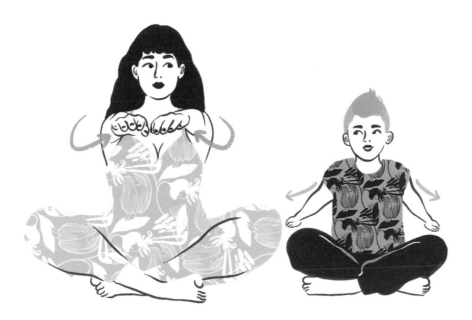

9. Fairy wings front and back

Sitting in yogi pose, hold your arms out straight in front of you. Breathe in.

As you breathe out, move your arms backwards.

Repeat this movement at least 10 times in time with your breath.

10. Fairy wings to the side

Sit in yogi pose, facing each other. Hold your arms out in front of you. Breathe in.

As you breathe out, turn your upper body and your head, and lift your arms up to one side. Your pelvis should stay on the floor. Breathe in and come back to the centre.

Breathe out and do the same on the other side.

Repeat this movement at least 10 times in time with your breath.

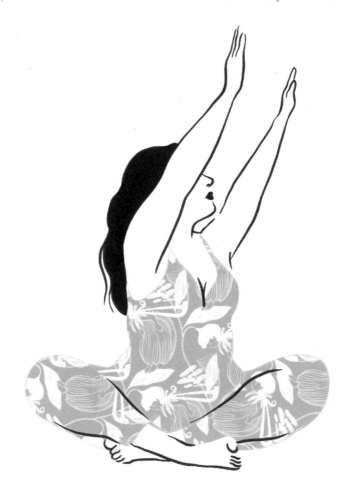

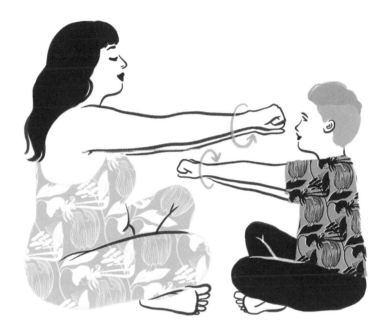

11. Small fairy arm rotations

Sit in yogi pose, facing each other. Hold out your arms in front of you, hands clenched.

Draw little circles in front of you in one direction with your outstretched arms.

Repeat this movement at least 10 times in time with your breath.

Then change direction.

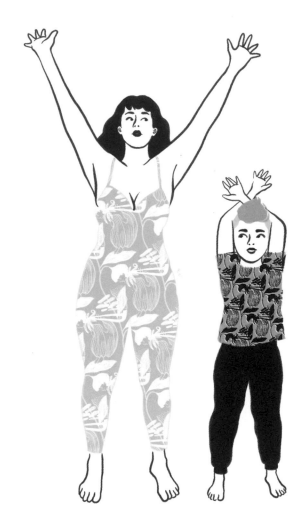

12. Big fairy parade

Stand up, facing each other with your feet hip-width apart.

Hold your hands up towards the sky to make a big V with them. Your fingers should be spread out. Breathe in.

As you breathe out, cross your arms above your head, keeping your arms straight.

Breathe in and bring your arms back to the big V.

Repeat this movement at least 10 times in time with your breath.

13. Fairy whirl

Stand up, back to back, with a bit of space between you, legs spread out roughly the width of your hips. Hold your arms out horizontally at your sides.

Breathe in and rotate your upper body, head and arms to the left and behind you. Your feet should stay flat on the floor.

Breathe out and turn to the right.

Repeat this whirling movement at least 10 times in time with your breath

While you rotate backwards to the left or right, you can try to touch the other person's hand.

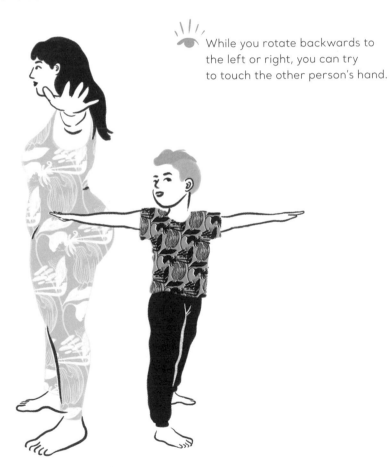

14. Standing fairy spreads wing to the side

Stand up, back to back, with a bit of space between you, legs spread out roughly the width of your hips. Hold your arms upwards.

Breathe in, turn your upper body and your head, with your arms moving in the same direction. Your feet should stay flat on the floor.

Breathe out and change sides without lowering your arms.

Repeat this movement at least 10 times in time with your breath.

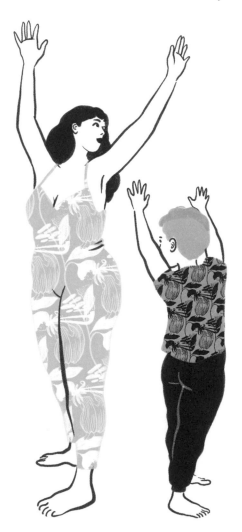

After spreading their wings, the fairy has fun taking a nice bow!

15. Fairy bow

Stand up straight, facing each other, legs apart.

Hold your arms out horizontally to the side. Breathe in.

As you breathe out, place your right hand on your left foot. Your left hand should point up towards the sky.

Breathe in and come back up to the pose with your arms straight out at your sides.

As you breathe out, do the same pose with the other hand.

Repeat this movement at least 10 times in time with your breath.

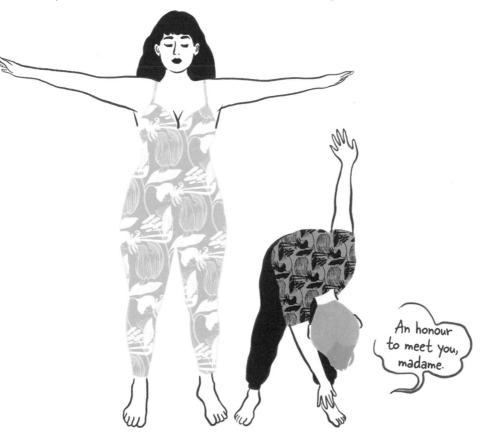

An honour to meet you, madame.

16. A visit from his friend the eagle

Stand with your weight on your left foot and bend your left knee to let your right leg wrap around the left, so one thigh is in front of the other.

If you can, curl your right foot around your left calf.

Lift your arms out by your sides to make big eagle wings – and fly!

As you breathe in, lift your arms up and as you breathe out lower them.

Then change legs.

 Suggestions for a more difficult pose:

If your balance permits, you can also entwine your arms. When you are standing on your left leg, hold your right arm bent in front of you and curl your left arm around it so your hands meet in front of your face.

Keep a balance between your arms and legs to stay stable as you try to keep your elbows and knees on the same line!

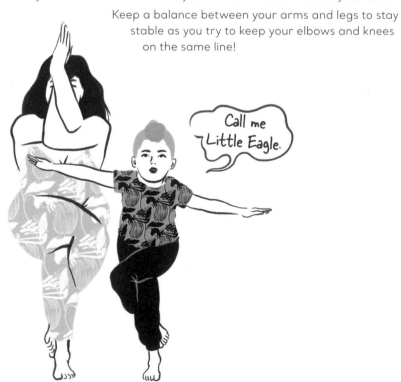

Call me Little Eagle.

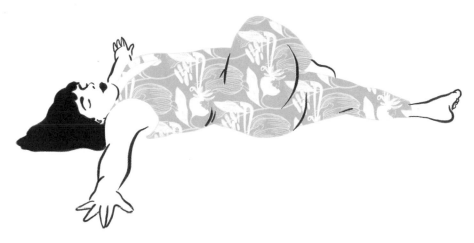

17. Lying down fairy twist

Lie down on your back, arms out on the floor to form a cross.

Bend your right leg up towards your chest and fold it over to the left side, with your left leg flat on the floor. Your shoulders should both stay on the floor and your head should face to the right.

Take a few breaths in this position, then change sides.

18. Relaxation

And now, time for relaxation (for guided relaxation, see page 28).

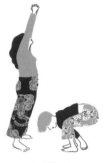

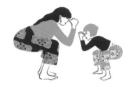

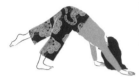

1. Elephant greeting with swinging trunks

2. Elephant greeting with trunks to the front

3. Elephant walks on its back feet

4. Elephant walks on all fours

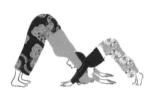

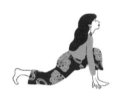

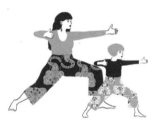

5. Elephant body stretch

6. Elephant stretch on one knee

7. Elephant learns archery

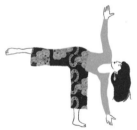

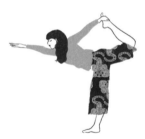

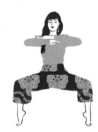

8. Elephant side balance

9. Elephant learns a dance move

10. Elephant imitates rugby players with a haka

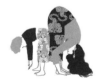

11. Head down elephant

12. Elephant fold

13. Relaxation

The elephant

For all ages
For all levels
For any time of day, apart from the evening
Duration: 20 to 25 minutess

This dynamic session lets you work on your grounding, sense of self-movement and body position, and general body mobility.
It's recommended if you need to use up some of your boundless energy, so avoid practising it in the evening.

Today we are taking a trip to Africa to watch a lovely herd of elephants!

1. Elephant greeting with swinging trunks

Stand face to face on the edge of your mats. Your feet should be hip-width apart, arms down beside your body, which should be nice and straight. Tense your legs, feet anchored to the floor and toes curled. Your legs are as strong as an elephant's!

Join your hands in front of you and cross your fingers over each hand, then lift them up to the level of your face – that's your elephant trunk!

As you breathe in, lift your arms above your head, keeping your fingers crossed.

Breathe out and bend your knees, but keep your feet in position, and bring your arms down between your knees. Swing your arms between your legs a few times, keeping your head fully relaxed. Then, as you breathe in, stand up again with your arms above your head.

Repeat this sequence at least three more times.

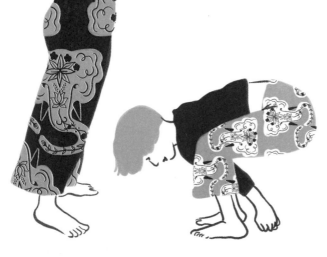

2. Elephant greeting with trunks to the front

Stand up facing each other. Spread your legs so they are a little wider than hip-width apart. Join your hands in front of you and cross your fingers over each hand, then lift them up to the level of your face – that's your elephant trunk!

As you breathe in, bend your knees so your upper body is parallel to the floor and greet each other with your trunks facing each other.

Take a few breaths in this pose. Then, as you breathe out, bring your body up and straighten your legs.

Start again and do this sequence at least three times.

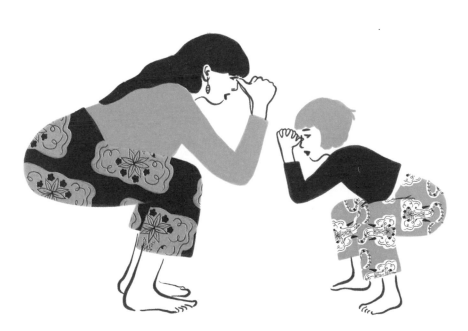

Now they have said hello, the elephants go for a walk together on the savannah.

3. Elephant walks on its back feet

Stand up facing each other. Bend forwards and grasp your ankles with your hands.

Look in front of you and, without bending your knees, move around the room in the style of an elephant, with big, heavy legs.

You can make a game of this, where you and your child try to touch each other with your heads while you're in this pose.

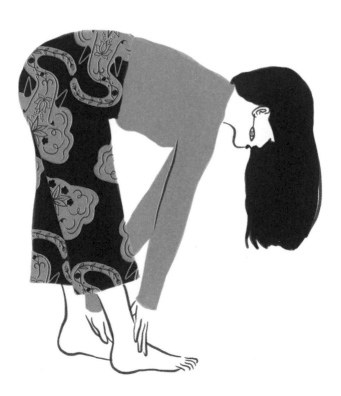

4. Elephant walks on all fours

Stand up facing each other, then bend forwards and put your hands and feet flat on the floor.

Take a big step backwards with your feet. Your hips should stay up, to form an upside-down V with your body.

Your hands should be shoulder-width apart with your fingers spread out, facing the front. Your knees should be hip-width apart.

Push hard with your hands, keeping your shoulders relaxed, and look forwards.

Look in front of you and move around the room in the style of an elephant, with big, heavy legs.

To move around, lift your right foot and right hand at the same time, and do the same on the other side.

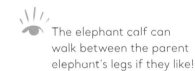
The elephant calf can walk between the parent elephant's legs if they like!

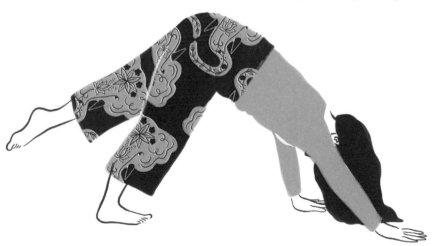

5. Elephant body stretch

Go back to the starting position of the inverted V on page 145.

From this position, make a big stretch by pushing your hands and feet, and tensing your arms and legs as much as you can. Push your hips up to the sky!

From here, lift one arm and then the other, then one leg and then the other, to feel the different stretches on each limb.

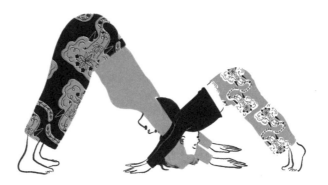

6. Elephant stretch on one knee

From the last position, take a deep breath in and place your left foot between your hands.

As you breathe out, lower your right knee to the floor, and raise your upper body and head to look straight in front of you. Breathe gently in this pose.

Come back to the inverted V and change legs.

If you're comfortable in this pose, raise your arms straight above your head!

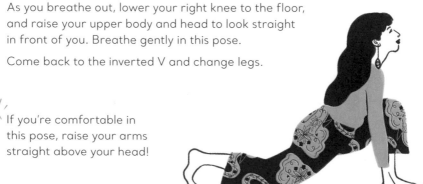

Now they've had a good stretch, the elephants are going to try some other activities.

7. Elephant learns archery

Stand up facing each other.

Take a big step back with your right foot and turn your left foot to face the front of your mat.

Raise your arms to shoulder height and make an archer's movement with your right arm. Aim at different places by moving your arms and your upper body, but don't move your legs.

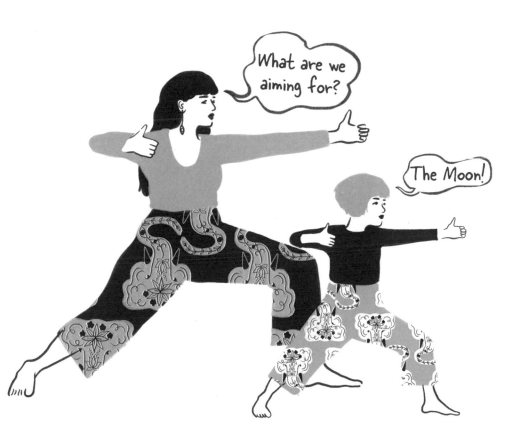

8. Elephant side balance

Stand up facing each other. Take a big step back with your right foot.

Lean forwards and put your left hand on the floor, bending your left knee. Slowly raise your right leg to the rear, up to the height of your hips. Raise your right arm, keeping it straight and turn your right hip up towards the sky. Keep your balance as you breathe. Gradually straighten your left leg. Look first at the floor, but then, if your balance allows, look to the right.

Put your right leg back and return to the front of the mat to change legs.

Help your child by holding their leg in the air so they can move their hips. When their right leg is in the air the entire hip should face the right side.

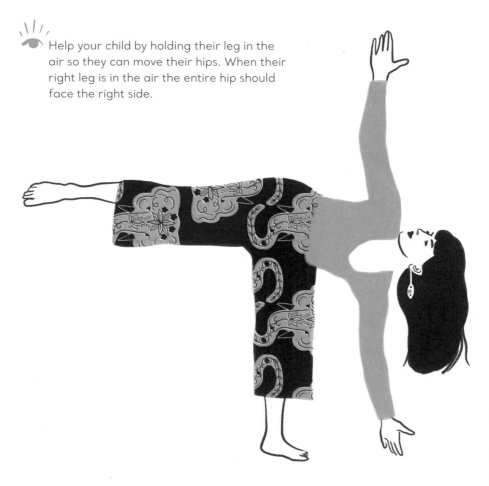

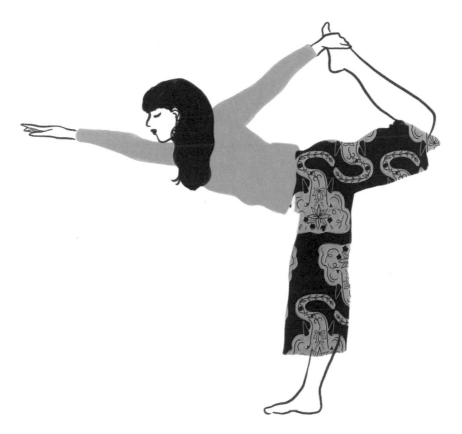

9. Elephant learns a dance move

Facing each other, stand on your right leg, swing your left leg behind you and, as you bend your knee, grasp your left foot with your left hand.

Hold on to each other with your right hands outstretched in front of you.

As you breathe in, raise your left leg by pushing gently with the foot against the hand.

Stand up gradually, in your own time, making sure your body does not lean forwards. Keep your body as straight as possible without forcing.

Breathe as you hold this pose.

Then, as you breathe out, place your left foot back on the floor and change sides.

10. Elephant imitates rugby players with a haka

Stand facing each other with your legs spread out wide.

Bend your knees and lift up as high as you can on your toes.

Lift your arms up straight to shoulder height in front of you and bend your elbows to lift your hands upwards. Then slap your right hand on to your left arm, and vice versa!

You can invent a shout together, for fun or, depending on how you're feeling, to cry out as you make this pose!

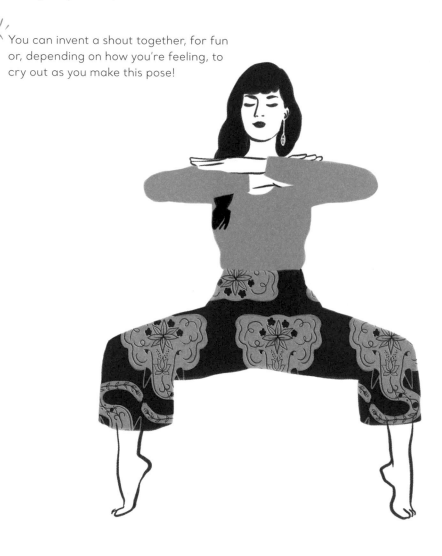

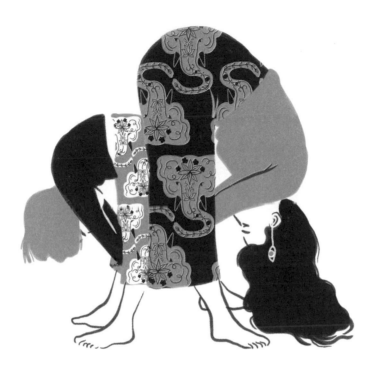

11. Head down elephant

Stand up back to back and spread your legs wide apart.

Put your hands on your hips. As you breathe in, bend forwards, keeping your back as straight as possible, and let your hands fall to the floor. Look at each other upside-down. Get your head down as close as you can to the floor. Your legs should be straight and your feet should be well anchored to the floor.

Hold each other's hands between your legs to help you stretch the upper back.

Breathe as you hold this pose.

Then let go of each other's hands and return to an upright position, keeping your back straight.

Go back to the front of your mat.

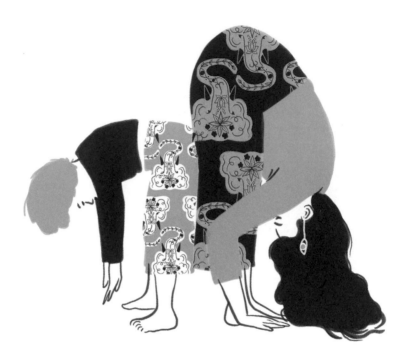

12. Elephant fold

For the forward fold, stand up straight, back to back, at the front of your mats.

Take a deep breath and as you breathe out lower yourself forwards, down towards your feet, with arms outstretched and back straight. When you're down, relax your back and arms to let your hands touch the floor.

If this stretch is too much, bend your knees so you can put your hands on your ankles or shins, wherever it's comfortable.

Breathe as you hold this pose.

Then bend your knees and sit down on your mat.

For the sitting fold, sit down with your legs in front of you.

Stretch up with your back and, as you breathe in, lift both arms up to the sky. Then, as you exhale, fold forwards gently and grasp your big toes, reaching round them with your index finger, middle finger and thumb of each hand.

Stay in this position and concentrate on your long, deep breathing.

Start with the lower back, then continue to bend, keeping your spine long. Your head bends over last.

If you or your child are unable to grip your big toes, bend forwards and hold on to whatever you can (ankles, calves, knees). Keep a straight back and stretch your legs.

To start with, show this pose to your child. Then do it with them, making sure they keep their back straight. Try it facing each other with your feet touching.

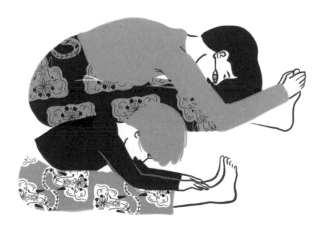

13. Relaxation

And now, time for relaxation (for guided relaxation, see page 28).

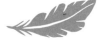

1. Duck walk

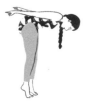

2. Duck does yogi squats

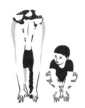

3. Duck stretches its wings

4. Duck stretches its feet

5. Duck dive

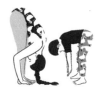

6. Frog pose

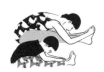

7. Frog jump

8. Frog stretch

9. Forward frog fold

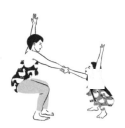

10. Sitting frog fold

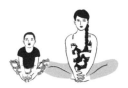

11. The butterfly

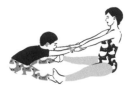

12. Butterfly plays with its wings

13. Butterfly stretches its wings

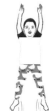

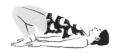

14. Half-bridge

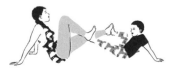

15. The pedalo

16. The happy child

17. Relaxation

The duck

For all ages
For all levels
For any time of day, apart from the evening
Duration: 20 to 25 minutes

Today we're going for a walk around a lovely lake where
ducks live with their friends, the frogs and butterflies!
This dynamic sequence is suitable for all, big and small.
It focuses on opening out the hips and strengthening legs.
It's recommended for the morning or afternoon.

As we arrive at the lake, we can see the ducks walking around, one behind the other. Let's do as they do!

1. Duck walk

Crouch down, one behind the other, heels wide apart.

To start with, keep your heels on the floor and put your hands together as if in prayer in front of your chest.

Your bent elbows should be next to your body like a duck's wings.

Now walk around the room like ducks, hands apart and heels up so you can move quite easily!

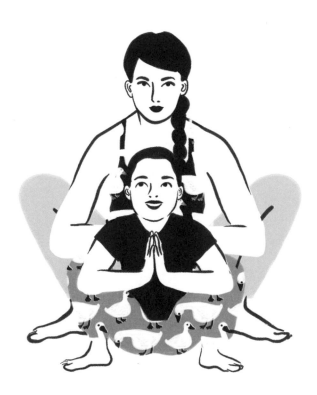

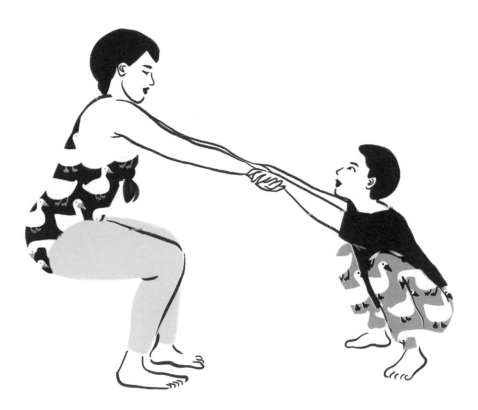

2. Duck does yogi squats

Crouch down facing each other and hold each other's hands.

Work together to balance, keeping your feet apart and, if possible, your heels on the floor.

This exercise is often easier for children than it is for parents.

Find the leg distance that works best for you: some people find yogi squats easy with their feet together, others don't. Everyone has a different level of flexibility.

Once you have both found a comfortable pose, test out how effective it is by letting go of each other's hands. If you fall over, start again!

Stay in this position and breathe.

In order to learn to swim well, the duck needs to strengthen its thighs by doing squats.

3. Duck stretches its wings

Staying in the yogi squat pose, hold each other with your left hands only. As you breathe in, stretch your right arm as high as you can towards the sky, keep your balance and look up towards your right hand.

As you breathe out, lower your arm and grip each other's right hands in front of you.

Then do the same movement with your left arm.

Repeat three times on each side.

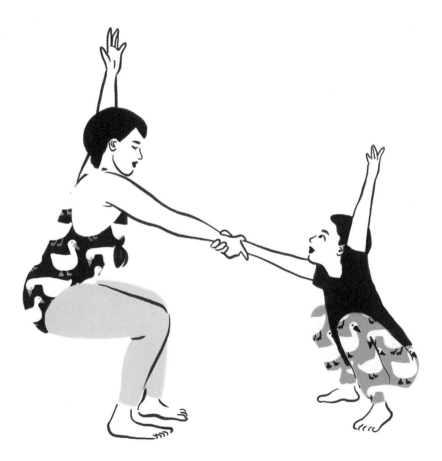

4. Duck stretches its feet

Stay in the yogi squat pose, and put your hands on the floor.

Straighten out your left leg in front of you as you breathe in, then fold it back under your body as you breathe out.

Then change sides. Repeat the movement on each side three times.

Do the same thing, but this time straighten out your left leg to your left side, then your right leg to your right side. Repeat three times on each side.

Then straighten first one leg and then the other behind you. Repeat three times on each side.

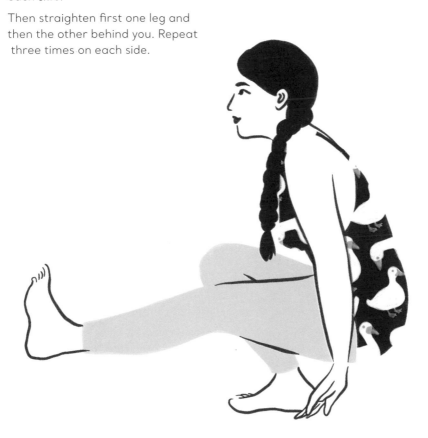

159

The ducks are going to splash around in the lake. To get into the water, they dive!

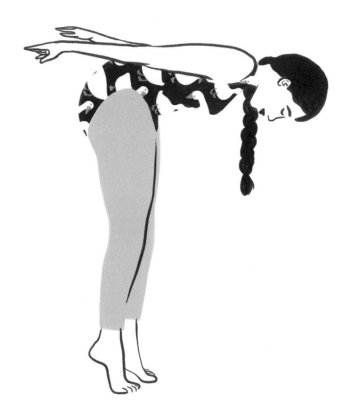

5. Duck dive

Stand up facing each other on the edge of your mats.

As you breathe in, rise up to stand on tiptoes and lean over forwards in order to make your body parallel with the floor. Hold your arms out behind you with your fingers spread out. Look at yourself!

When you exhale, lift your chest and bring the soles of your feet to the ground.

Repeat three times.

We have just seen some frogs who are playing at the edge of the lake. They are stretching their legs and jumping around!

6. Frog pose

Stand up facing each other with your feet together.

Crouch down on to your toes, keeping your heels together.

Place your hands between your knees and your fingers on the floor.

Keep your head up straight, look at each other.

Breathe in as you bring your hips upwards and lower your head, looking between your knees, always with your heels off the ground.

Breathe out and go back to the starting position, crouching down.

Do this movement five times.

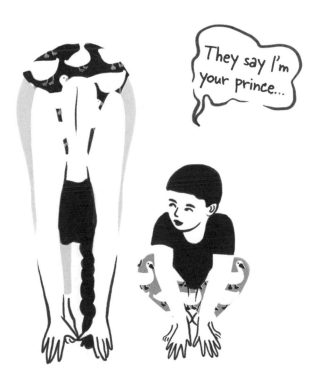

They say I'm your prince...

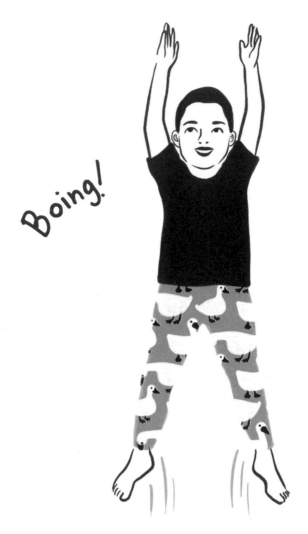

Boing!

7. Frog jump

Crouch down on your toes, with your heels together, as for frog pose

Place your hands between your knees, with your fingers touching the floor.

Keep your head up straight.

Jump forwards with a big push of the legs and move around the room like this.

8. Frog stretch

Get into the yogi squat pose (see 2, page 157) with your feet apart. Lean forwards so your back is parallel to the floor, keeping your spine straight. Place your arms below your thighs to put your hands flat on the back of your feet or your heels.

Look at the floor, then turn your head to the right as you breathe in and to the left as you breathe out.

Repeat the head movements five times.

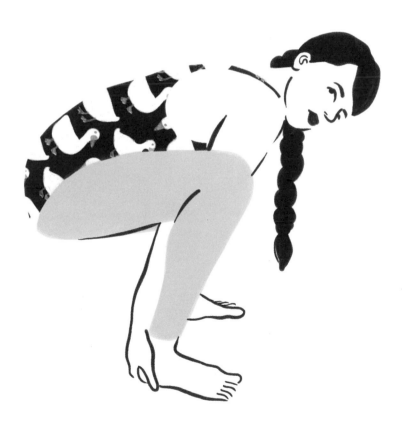

9. Forward frog fold

Stand up facing each other at the edge of your mats.

Take a deep breath and, as you breathe out, lower your body, arms outstretched and back straight, down towards your feet.

When you're down, relax your back and arms to put your hands flat on the floor. If this stretch is too much, bend your knees so you can put your hands on your ankles or shins, wherever it's comfortable. Breathe as you hold this pose.

Then bend your knees and sit down on your mat.

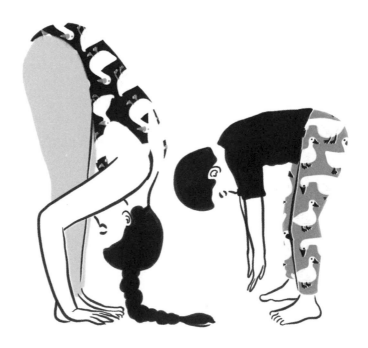

10. Sitting frog fold

Sit down facing each other with your legs out in front of you.

Straighten up your back and, as you breathe in, lift both arms up to the sky. Then, as you exhale, fold over forwards gently and grasp your big toes, reaching round them with your index finger, middle finger and thumb of each hand.

Stay in this position and concentrate on your long, deep breathing.

Start with the lower back and then your body, keeping your spine elongated. Your head bends over last.

If you or your child are unable to grip your big toes, bend forwards and hold on to whatever you can (ankles, calves, knees). Keep a straight back and stretch your legs.

 To start with, get into this pose and show your child. Then do it with them, making sure they keep their back straight. Then you can do it together. Try it facing each other with your feet touching. If you are supple enough, hold on to each other's hands!

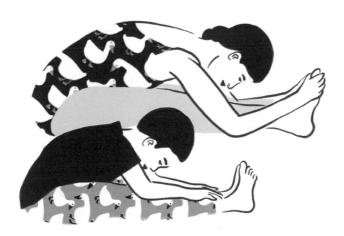

11. The butterfly

Sit down with your back straight. Place the soles of your feet together and wrap your hands around your feet.

In this pose you are going to flap your butterfly wings by moving your knees up and down vigorously.

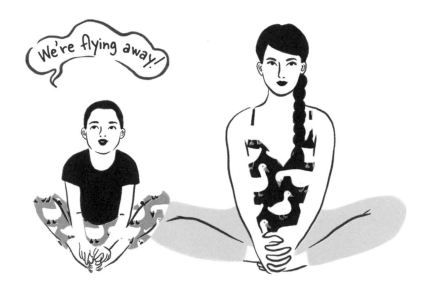

We're flying away!

This butterfly needs to build up their strength.

Stay in this position with your knees towards the floor. Stretch upwards with your back as if you're drinking water that's rolling off a leaf.

As you breathe out, bend forwards, keeping your back straight, and bring your body as close as you can to the floor, so the butterfly can drink the nectar from the flowers. Breathe in as you move back up and flap your wings again.

Repeat these stretches a few times to give your little butterfly plenty to eat and drink.

12. Butterfly plays with its wings

From the butterfly pose, lift up your bent right leg in front of you and hold your right foot with your left hand and put your right hand on your right knee.

Rock the leg by pulling your foot towards you and pushing your knee away from you, then by pushing your foot away from you as you pull your knee towards you.

After this pose, relax your left hand and place it on the floor.

Take your right foot in your right hand and bring your foot towards your ear as if you were making a telephone call with it!

Let go of your right leg and change sides.

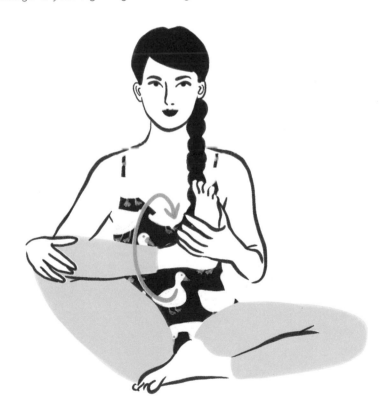

167

13. Butterfly stretches its wings

Sit facing each other with your legs apart. If you're able to, put your feet together. Otherwise, place the feet of your child on your calves.

Take hold of each other's hands with your arms straight in front of you. Lean forwards, keeping your back straight as you breathe in, and try to get your face all the way down to the floor.

Do the same movement to the right, then the left, getting your face down to your legs on one side and then the other.

Come back to the centre.

Then one of you leans back, pulling the other one gently forwards like like a pendulum movement. Then change sides.

Do these movements in a fluid, dynamic manner.

Open your legs progressively wider, making sure you do not overstretch the muscles in your legs and your lower back.

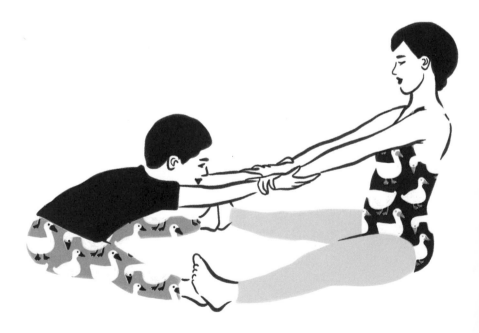

We are going to cross over a bridge to get to the other side of the lake.

14. Half-bridge

Lie on your backs side by side. Put your feet flat on the floor just in front of your buttocks.

Bend your knees and hold on to your ankles with your hands. Then, as you breathe in, lift your hips towards the sky as high as you can, but without lifting your upper back or your head. Concentrate on opening out your ribcage.

As you breathe out lower yourself down, vertebra by vertebra, from the centre of your back, then your lower back and finally your hips.

Repeat this movement three times.

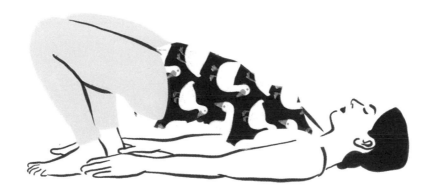

Show this pose to your child first and ask them to move some of their stuffed toys around under your back as if it were a bridge. Then swap roles.

We are going for a trip on the lake in a pedalo – lucky us!

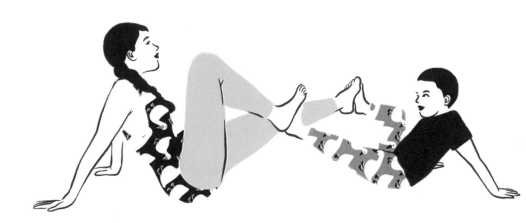

15. The pedalo

Sit facing each other. Place your hands on the floor behind you and keep your arms straight. Put the soles of your feet together, push your feet one by one, and pedal!

16. The happy child

Lie on your back and bend your legs with your knees apart. Put your arms between your legs and grab the outsides of your feet. Your head should be resting on your mat.

Bring your knees down towards the floor.

Breathe deeply in this pose for a dozen respiratory cycles and then tip your body weight from one side to the other, as if giving yourself a back massage!

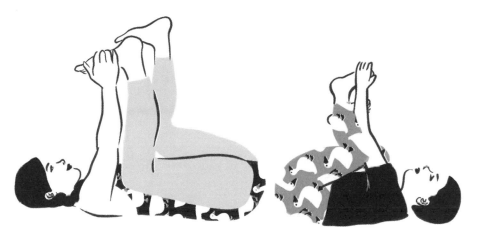

17. Relaxation

And now, time for relaxation (for guided relaxation, see page 28).

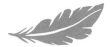

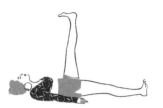

1. Grasshopper lifts one leg

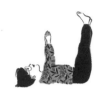

2. Grasshopper lifts two legs

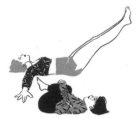

3. Grasshopper bends and stretches

4. Grasshopper backwards leg stretch

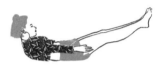

5. Grasshopper stretch pose

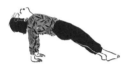

6. Grasshopper backwards bend

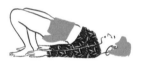

7. Grasshopper half-bridge

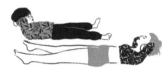

8. Grasshopper abs stretch with legs apart

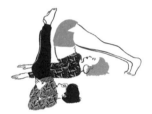

9. Grasshopper and the candle

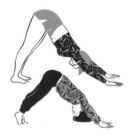

10. Downward-facing dog

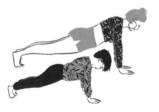

11. Dog plank

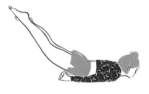

12. Grasshopper pose

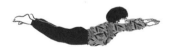

13. Grasshopper stretches

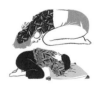

14. Forward stretches from knee sitting position

15. Relaxation

The grasshopper

From six years
For all levels
For any time of day, apart from the evening
Duration: 25 to 30 minutes

This sequence is designed to strengthen your abdominal wall.

It's dynamic and can be done in the morning or afternoon with children aged six years and over.

To start with, hold the poses for a short time only. Then you can progressively increase the length you hold them for, depending on the age of your child and how often you practise.

Today we're going to spend some time with a family of very clever grasshoppers! Grasshoppers use their legs a lot and we're going to watch and copy them.

1. Grasshopper lifts one leg

Sit down facing each other with your legs out in front of you on your mat, your feet at the edge and the soles of your feet facing, but not touching. Then lie on your back, your hands below your hips, palms firmly on the floor. Breathe in as you lift your right leg to a 90-degree angle.

Breathe out as you slowly lower your straightened leg to the floor.

Do the same thing with your left leg.

Continue to alternate between right and left legs.

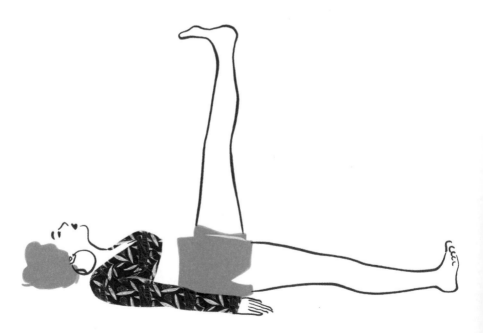

2. Grasshopper lifts two legs

Lying on your back, lift both arms straight up to the sky so they are at 90 degrees. Keep them like this for the entire exercise.

As you breathe in, lift both of your feet to an angle of 90 degrees. As you breathe out, lower your legs down to the floor.

Keep both of your arms pointing upwards at a 90-degree angle for the whole time.

As you do this pose, if your back arches or you are in pain, put your hands or a small cushion under your hips.

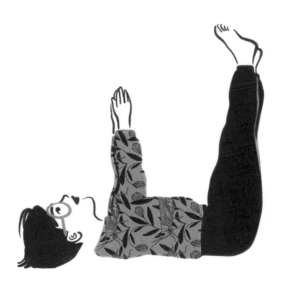

3. Grasshopper bends and stretches

Lying on your back, bend your knees and bring them to your chest. Wrap your arms around them, with your head lying on the floor.

Breathe in and move your arms out to your sides and on to the floor, and move your legs straight out in front of you at an angle of 60 degrees to the floor.

Breathe out and come back to the starting position.

Repeat this movement at least five times.

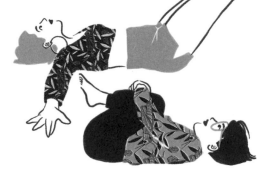

4. Grasshopper backwards leg stretch

Lying on your back, bend your left knee and wrap your arms around it, with your head lying on the floor. Breathe in and lift your right leg straight up at an angle of 90 degrees to the floor. Breathe out and lower the straight leg to the floor.

Do this movement 10 times. Then change legs.

As the grasshoppers do their leg movements while lying on their backs, they see something flying through the sky, so they stop and stretch without moving to take a look.

5. Grasshopper stretch pose

Lie down on your backs facing each other with your feet together. Your lower back should be in contact with the floor.

Hold out your arms and hands, palms facing, towards your hips (on the side or above).

Lift the top of your ribcage, then your head and look at your toes, which should be hiding your partner's face. Lift your feet to 15cm from the floor.

Stay in this position and breathe slowly and deeply.

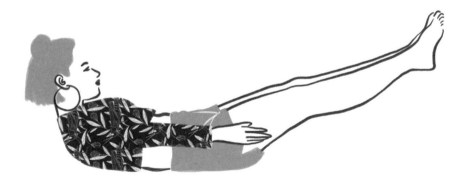

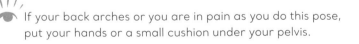 If your back arches or you are in pain as you do this pose, put your hands or a small cushion under your pelvis.

The grasshoppers move slowly and stretch their tummies towards the sky. Let's do the same.

6. Grasshopper backwards bend

Sit down with your legs out in front of you. Place your hands flat on the floor behind you with your fingers pointing in the direction of your toes.

Raise your chest and hips. Tilt your head backwards without letting it fall right back and push your ribcage up towards the sky.

Your heels and toes should remain on the floor and your body should be as straight as possible.

Stay in this position and breathe in and out at least three times.

If your neck is delicate, it's better to keep your head straight at the top of your body and your chin close to your throat.

To start with you can show this pose to your child, who can have fun making toys go underneath or using your body as a giant slide for the toys. Then, help your child get into position so they can have a turn at making a lovely slide for their toys.

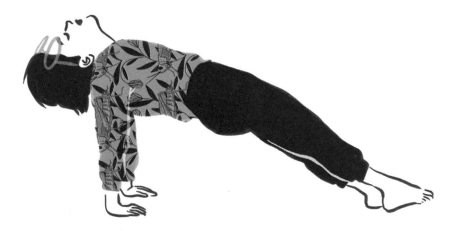

The grasshoppers continue their exercises.

7. Grasshopper half-bridge

Lie on your back. Bend your knees. Your feet should be flat on the floor. Hold your ankles.

Breathe in, contract your abs and lift your pelvis.

Concentrate on opening out your ribcage. Keep your head on the floor and bring your shoulder blades together for a more intense opening of the ribcage. Breathe deeply in this position. Breathe out and, vertebra by vertebra, bring your back down to the floor, using your thighs and muscles in your buttocks.

Continue to alternate the movements.

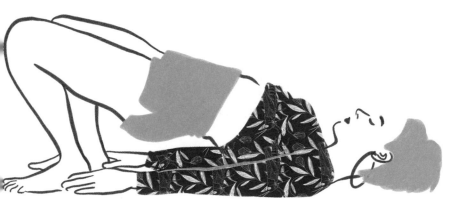

In order to jump a long way, grasshoppers need strong abdominals. They have a strange way of training, though!

8. Grasshopper abs stretch with legs apart

Sit face to face with your feet touching each other.

Lie down on your back with your legs apart, straight out along the floor. Put your hands on your shoulders and breathe in. As you breathe out slowly, lift up your torso until you're sitting up and then clap your hands together with your partner. Breathe in and go back to the starting position.

As you breathe out slowly, lift up and lean towards your right leg, keeping your hands on your shoulders.

Breathe in and come back to the lying down starting position.

As you breathe out slowly, lift up and lean towards your left leg, keeping your hands on your shoulders.

Continue like this by alternating forwards, right and left, each time coming back to the lying down starting position.

You can choose to keep the same order (forward, right, left) each time, or vary it.

For a change, you can select one of you to decide the order and the other one has to follow them. Then change the leader.

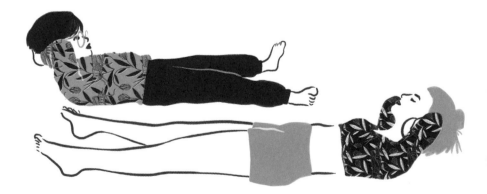

9. Grasshopper and the candle

Lie on your back with your arms beside your body, palms down.

Raise your legs to 90 degrees from the floor. Lift your pelvis up to get into candle pose. Put your hands on your lower back, elbows on the floor.

Take long, deep breaths to help you stay in this position.

For the youngest ones, or children who aren't used to this, help them to start by lifting their legs and holding them as straight as possible. Also help them to get out of this position by carefully unrolling them back.

Women shouldn't do this pose if they are pregnant or at the start of their menstrual cycle.

Next, gently move your straight legs behind your head.

Stay in this position and, if you can, put your toes on the floor. Breathe.

Then stay in this pose and spread your legs. Breathe.

Bring your legs back together and bend your knees in order to get them as close as you can to your ears.

To get out of this position, keep your knees bent and gently bring your legs back in front of you. Stay lying down for a little while.

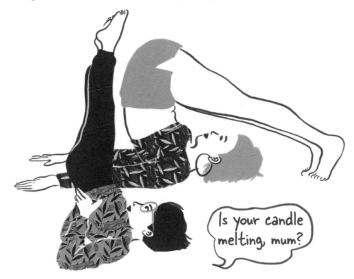

Is your candle melting, mum?

A dog is passing by and has seen the grasshopper family doing their exercises. He wants to say hello and praise the grasshoppers for their skills. Let's copy the dog!

10. Downward-facing dog

Get on to all fours.

Bend forwards, and place your hands and feet flat on the floor, your pelvis in the air so you make an upside-down V-shape with your body.

Your hands should be shoulder-width apart and your fingers should be spread out and pointing forwards. Your knees should be the same width apart as your hips.

Push down hard with your hands, shoulders relaxed, head tucked in, and look at your belly button.

Start with your toes on the floor. Then bend your right knee and stretch your left leg, lowering your left heel to the floor. Do the same on the other side and repeat this a few times. If you can, have both heels on the floor.

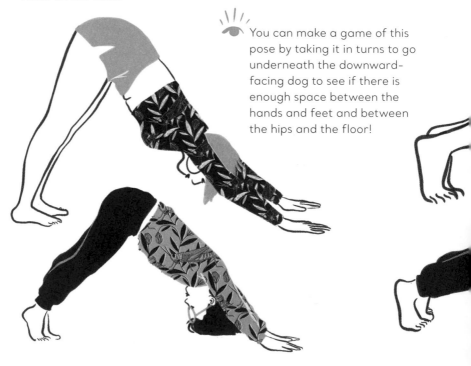

You can make a game of this pose by taking it in turns to go underneath the downward-facing dog to see if there is enough space between the hands and feet and between the hips and the floor!

Then the dog proudly shows off his plank position.

11. Dog plank

Lying on your front, place your hands flat on the floor.

Lift yourself off the floor by straightening your arms. Heels up, with the tops of your feet on the floor. Keep your head straight at the top of your spine. The body should be in a straight line from your neck to your feet. Help yourself to stay in this pose by breathing in and out deeply.

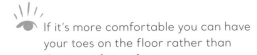 If it's more comfortable you can have your toes on the floor rather than the tops of your feet.

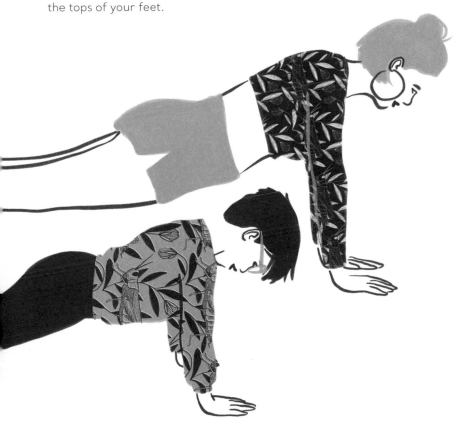

Intrigued, the grasshopper family stay still and watch the dog.

12. Grasshopper pose

Lie face-down on the floor, feet together.

Place your hands in fists under your pelvis where your thighs meet your hips. Pushing down with your fists, lift your right leg, keeping your left leg on the floor.

Change legs.

Then, lift both legs in the air and tense the back of your thighs to keep your legs stretched.

Use your fists to lift your legs from the hips.

Keep your chin on the floor.

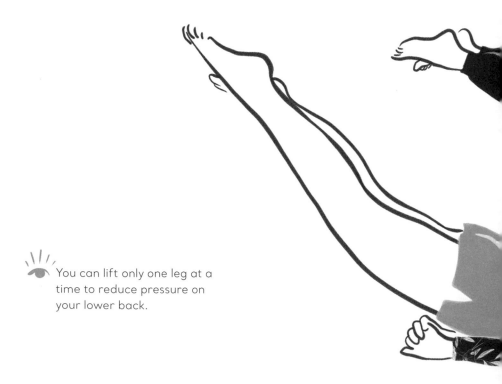

You can lift only one leg at a time to reduce pressure on your lower back.

Grasshopper stretches out their front and back legs.

13. Grasshopper stretches

Lie on your front, with arms out and up in front of you, palms together.

With your legs tensed and together, contract your upper thigh muscles and lift your legs up.

Make a big stretch in your lower back – imagine that you're being lifted up by the toes, causing a stretch in the lower back. Only your belly button should be touching the floor.

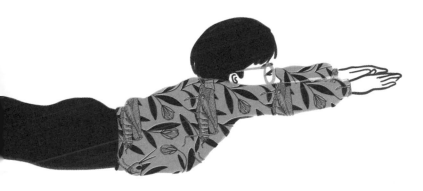

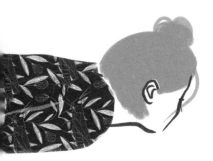

> In order to say goodbye, the grasshopper family greets us by bending forwards.

14. Forward stretches from knee sitting position

Get down on your knees and sit on your heels.

Your fingers should be crossed in the Venus lock 'mudra', at the back of the neck.

To do the Venus lock 'mudra' cross all of your fingers, but differently depending on whether you are a boy/man or a girl/woman. A man or boy should have their left little finger at the bottom and the left thumb between the right thumb and index finger. A woman or girl should have the right little finger at the bottom and the right thumb between the left index finger and thumb.

You have to do it to understand the subtle difference!

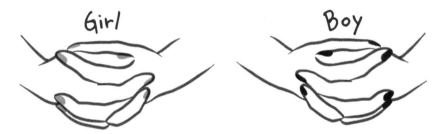

Breathe in and, as you breathe out, lean forwards to put your forehead on the floor. Your buttocks should stay on your heels.

Breathe in and straighten up, then continue the movement.

When you have finished this pose you can sit up with your legs out in front of you, shaking them out and massaging them.

As you leaning forwards, if you or your child are unable to reach the floor with your forehead you can put a cushion in front of you and rest on that.

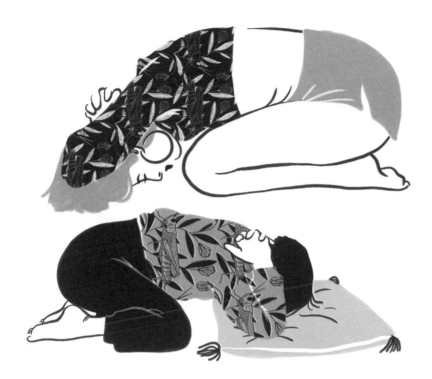

15. Relaxation

And now for some relaxation
(for guided relaxation, see page 28).

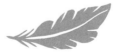

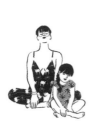 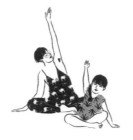 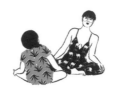

1. The camel walk   2. The sitting puppet   3. The mixing spoon   4. The cat

 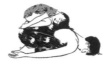 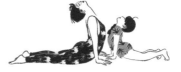

5. The camel   6. Child's pose   7. The cobra

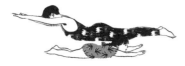 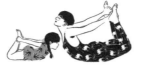 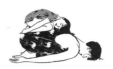

8. Supermen and superwomen of the desert   9. The bow   10. Child's pose

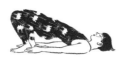 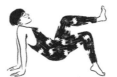 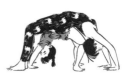

11. The little bridge   12. The bridge   13. The spider   14. The big wheel

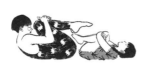 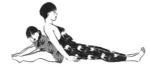 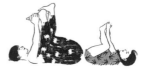

15. The ball   16. The scales   17. The happy child

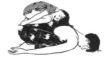

18. Child's pose   19. Relaxation

The camel

From six years
Advanced level
For any time of day, apart from the evening
Duration: 25 to 30 minutes

Today we're going to the desert to meet a caravan of camels.
This session concentrates on the opening out of the back and
improving its suppleness.
This is an invigorating sequence.

To help with suppleness of our backs, we are going for a walk on a camel's back – off we go!

1. The camel walk

Before we leave for the camel walk it's important to be sitting properly.

Sit in yogi pose and hold your ankles with your hands.

Breathe in deeply to fill your belly, arch your back, stomach out and head right up.

Breathe out deeply, round your back, bring your head down and look at your stomach.

Continue to alternate between these movements smoothly, like a wave coming and going on a beach.

When you can do the movement easily, go faster, but keep the smoothness of movement and do it in time with your breathing, listening carefully.

Breathe deeply, come back to your starting position and breathe out.

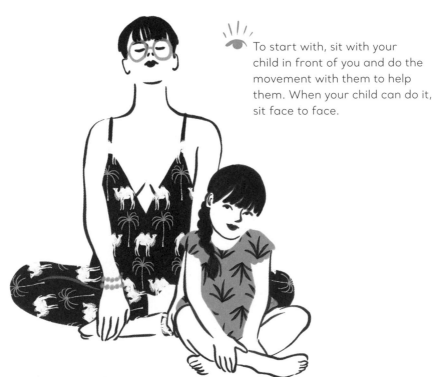

To start with, sit with your child in front of you and do the movement with them to help them. When your child can do it, sit face to face.

Now we've been for a ride on the back of a camel, let's pretend to be puppets.

2. The sitting puppet

Staying in yogi pose, put your hands on your hips, breathe in and lean over to your left. Breathe out and come back to the centre. Breathe in and lean over to your right. Then breathe out and come back to the centre. Carry on with a fluid movement, like a puppet!

Then put your right hand on the floor next to your pelvis, lift your left arm above your head and stretch your body over to the right. You should feel a stretch on your left side.

Then change sides.

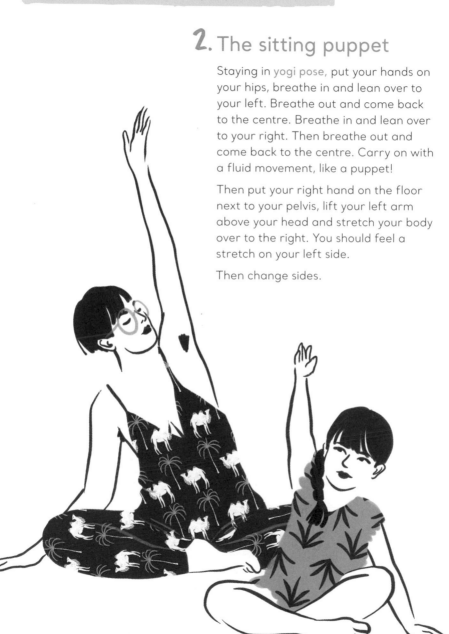

We've put up our shelter. Now it's time to stir the lovely dish that's cooking on the fire!

3 The mixing spoon

Start in the yogi pose. Place your hands on your knees.

Make big circles with your spine, breathing in as you lean forwards and breathing out as you lean backwards.

Your head should stay still, at the top of your shoulders. Your ribcage should remain open. Don't let your head drop forwards.

To start with, sit with your child in front of you and do the movement with them to help them. When your child can do it, sit face to face and do the movements together, mirroring each other and with the same rhythm.

When your faces meet, perhaps that's time for a kiss!

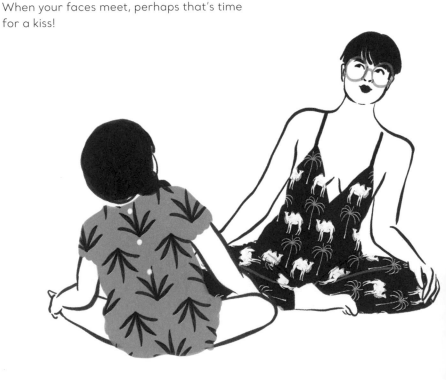

A cat approaches, attracted by the smell of food. Let's copy them!

4. The cat

Get on all fours. Place your hands on the floor, shoulder-width apart, with your fingers pointing forwards. Your knees should be the same width apart as your hips.

Breathe in, hollow your back and direct your buttocks towards the sky. Your head and neck should be stretched towards your back without straining them. Open out your ribcage and push your chin upwards and backwards, without relaxing your neck.

Then breathe out and round your back, direct your buttocks towards the floor and bring your chin towards your chest. Continue moving between the two poses in a fluid, regular manner. Move your lower back first, the upper back second and the head last.

Start slowly and when you have a good rhythm established you can speed up the movements. Alternate between the two positions as quickly as you feel, always being careful to move the head last.

Meow ♥

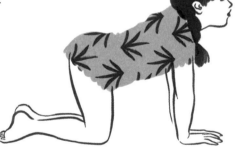

 To start with, you could show your child and ask them to put a soft toy on your back, to encourage them to take part and to see their toy go up and down with the rhythm of the movement. Then help your child to kneel next to you and do the pose with them. You can then put a soft toy on their back to see it go up and down with the movement.

When your child can do it well, face each other and do the movements together.

We've been watching the camels and imitating them, now we'll make some bends and curves with our bodies!

5. The camel

Get on your knees and sit down on your heels. The optimum space between your knees is roughly the width of two fists, side to side. Lift your pelvis and bring yourself up straight, staying on your knees. Your feet should be flat on the floor.

Feel your body rooted to the floor, from your knees.

Push your pelvis forwards and upwards, open out your ribcage towards the sky and breathe out as you lean back, placing your hands on your lower back and bringing your shoulder blades together. Then, if you can, hold your heels.

To start with, help your child to get into this pose slowly, then when they are able to do it well practise it together. To help you get used to this pose, you could start with your toes on the floor to raise your heels, if that makes it easier.

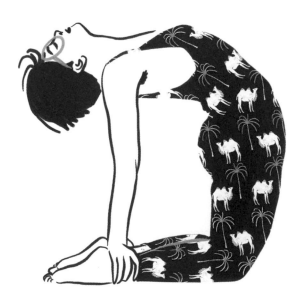

Now we've copied a camel's back, we're going
to have a rest in child's pose.

6. Child's pose

Get on your knees and sit on your heels. Lift your arms up in the air
and gently bring them down to the floor. Once your hands are down,
try to go as far forward as you can to really stretch out your back.
Count to 10. Without getting up, bring your arms backwards along
the length of your body to your feet and relax completely for a while
in this pose.

Breathe in your own rhythm.

To move out of this position, place your hands on the floor below your
shoulders and gently, moving from the bottom of your spine first, rise
up one vertebra at a time.

 For really small ones, and if it is OK for your back, your child can do
this pose on your back for relaxation.

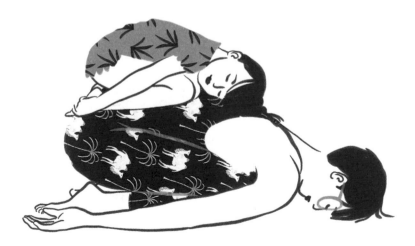

In the desert, we come across a family of cobras. Once they have left, let's see what it's like to be them.

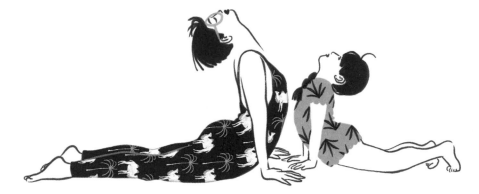

7. The cobra

To start with, we're going to be little cobras.

Lie down on your front facing each other. Your legs and your feet should be clenched. Place your hands below your shoulders, lift your chest and head up, keeping the palms of your hands flat on the floor. Your elbows should be next to your body.

Breathe in deeply and, as you breathe out, make a snake's hiss by sticking your tongue out a little. Hold the pose and have some fun.

After this, little cobras are going to grow and as they grow they lift up higher.

From the little cobra pose, breathe in and push with your hands so your arms are straight and helping to lift your chest and torso up further.

Make your spine stretch by opening out your ribcage, but be careful not to strain your lower back.

If it's too difficult to keep your arms straight, go back to the little cobra pose.

Don't lean too far backwards.

If you practise this pose you will gradually be able to stay in the full cobra pose for longer.

If you are unable to do this with your feet together, spread them out slightly, making sure the tops of your thighs stay in contact with the floor.

In the desert it turns out that we have superpowers! We're going to learn how to fly!

8. Supermen and superwomen of the desert

Lie down on the floor on your front, facing each other or side by side.

Your legs should be on the floor and your left arm on the floor next to your body with the hand in the direction of your feet, palm on the floor. Stretch out your right arm to the front and upwards, palm facing down, like Superman. Then change arms, and repeat five times.

Then lift both arms together. Count to 10. You can do this for longer as you progress.

Put your arms back on the floor in front of you and lift your right leg up, keeping it tense. Then change legs and repeat five times.

Then lift both legs together. Count to 10. Again, you can do this for longer as you progress.

Lower yourself down to the floor.

Lift and stretch your right leg and your left arm.

Then change over and stretch your left leg and your right arm. Alternate five times.

Now, are you ready to fly? Lift both arms and both legs at the same time! Count to 10. As before, you can do this for longer as you progress.

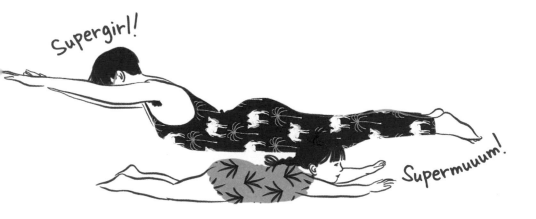

197

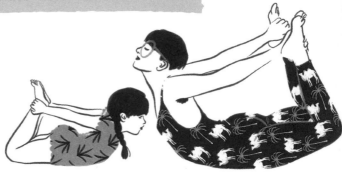

Now we're going to do some archery with the friends we have met in the desert!

9. The bow

Lie on your front, grab hold of your ankles and, using your thigh muscles, lift up your torso.

Then lift your legs upwards. Your head should be straight at the top of your body.

Your legs should be active, your ankles pushing into your hands and helping you to keep your arms straight behind you and keeping you up.

Have fun rocking back and forth, using your legs.

If you can, try to keep your big toes together. Your knees should be slightly apart.

Breathe in and out deeply. Use your breathing to help you stay in this pose.

10. Child's pose

Get on your knees and sit on your heels. Lift your arms up in the air and gently bring them down to the floor. Once your hands are down, try to go as far forward as you can to really stretch out your back. Count to 10. Without getting up, bring your arms backwards along the length of your body to your feet and relax completely for a while in this pose.

Breathe in your own rhythm.

To move out of this position, place your hands below your shoulders and gently, moving from the bottom of your spine first, rise up one vertebra at a time.

We can see a little bridge! Could there be some water around here?

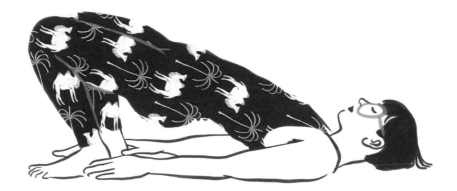

11. The little bridge

Lie on your back and bend your knees. Your feet should be flat on the floor. Hold on to your ankles.

Breathe in, contract your abs and lift your pelvis up. Concentrate on opening up your ribcage.

Breathe out and, vertebra by vertebra, lower your back down to the floor, using your thighs and your buttock muscles.

Continue to alternate up and down as you breathe in and out.

An oasis! There is water! The camels will be able to quench their thirst and rest. Let's cross over the big bridge to get to the oasis!

12. The bridge

Your body is going to make a bridge.

Sit down, legs out on the floor. Bend your knees with your feet flat on the floor, hip-width apart.

Place your arms behind your body, palms flat on the floor, fingers pointing in the direction of your feet. Lift your hips to make a nice, straight bridge.

Your chin should be in a straight line with your chest in order to keep your head in the same line as your body.

Use your breathing to help hold the pose.

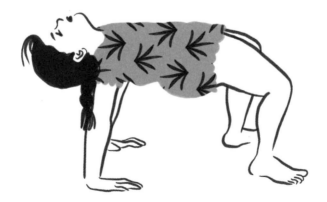

To start with, get your child into position and do it with them to help. You can make stuffed toys or cars go under the bridge.

Then you can get into position and your child can make sure that the bridge is nice and straight, and have fun going under it themselves!

In a corner of the oasis a group of spiders
is playing. Shall we copy them?

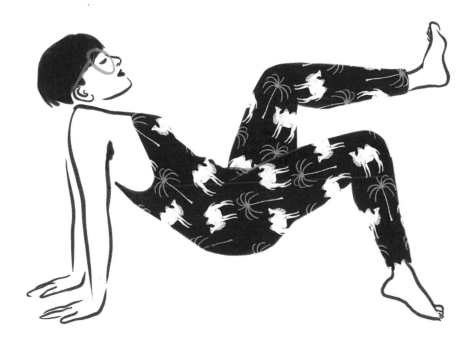

13. The spider

From the bridge pose, lower your pelvis without
touching the floor and walk around as you try to
touch each other with your big toes.

14. The big wheel

Lie on your back. Bend your knees and place your feet flat on the floor.

Place your hands flat on the floor very near your shoulders, with your fingers pointing towards your feet.

Breathe in and push with your hands and feet to bring your pelvis to the sky.

Breathe out and, if you can, breathe in and out twice in this position before you lower yourself down to the floor gently.

Help your child to get into this pose slowly. If they are unable to do it at first, stand them up against a wall, and lift their arms and place them behind their head, so the palms of the hands are flat on the wall. With the help of their hands, your child will be able to go down the wall a little, or all the way to the floor, depending on how supple they are. Help them by placing your hands on their lower back.

Then you can get into the pose and let your child have fun by going underneath.

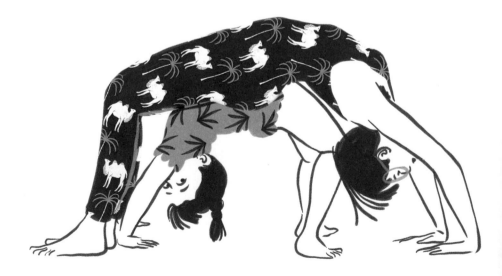

After they have stretched out their backs, the spiders relax by rolling into a ball!

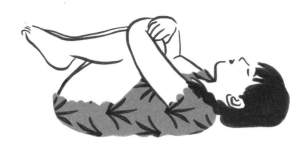

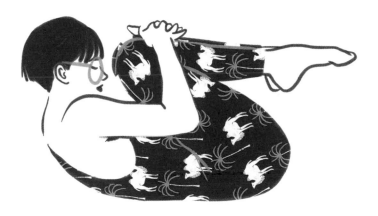

15. The ball

Lie on your back. Bring your knees up to your chest and wrap your arms around them. Massage your back by rocking backwards and forwards gently.

After that long walk in the desert, we're going to do some work to relax our backs!

16. The scales

Sit back to back. Your legs should be stretched out in front of you on the floor.

You should lean forwards, relaxing your whole body including your head. Your child should follow this movement by staying against your back, stretching themselves backwards towards you. Count to five and then lean the other way.

Your child leans forwards and relaxes and you tilt backwards. Count to five.

Then alternate, in a continuous movement, like a rocking horse.

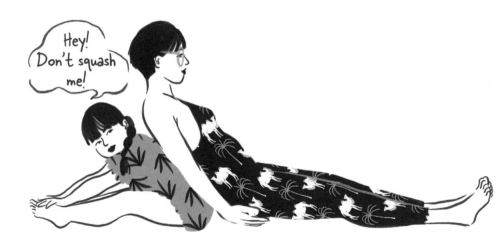

17. The happy child

Lie on your back, head on the floor. Bend your knees and reach your arms between your legs to hold on to the outside of your feet with your hands. Stay in this pose for five breaths in and out. Then, staying in this pose, ask your child to behave like a baby who has just woken up and started to move their legs, hands and body. Do the same yourself!

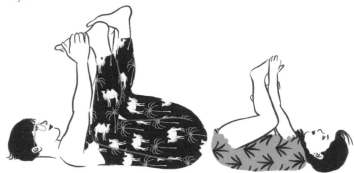

18. Child's pose

Get on your knees and sit down on your heels. Lift your arms up in the air and gently bring them down to the floor. Once your hands are down, try to go as far forward as you can to really stretch out your back. Count to 10. Without getting up, bring your arms backwards along the length of your body to your feet and relax completely for a while in this pose.

Breathe in your own rhythm.

To move out of this position, place your hands below your shoulders and gently, moving from the bottom of your spine first, rise up one vertebra at a time.

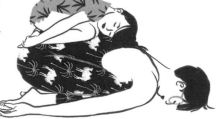

19. Relaxation

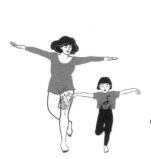

1. The flamingo

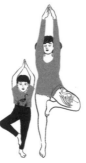

2. The flamingo's favourite tree

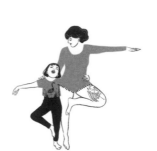

3. The mightiest tree in the forest

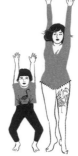

4. The palm tree

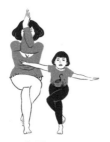

5. The eagle

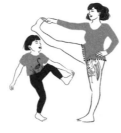

6. The leg game

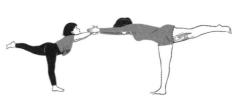

7. The warrior 3

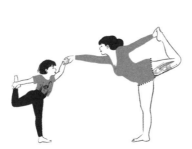

8. Supple like a flamingo

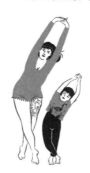

9. The flamingo's bow

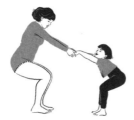

10. The flamingo in its chair

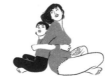

11. The roly-poly flamingo

12. Relaxation

The flamingo's day

From six years
Advanced level
For any time of day
Duration: 15 to 20 minutes

This sequence works on your balance, sense of movement and general muscle strength.
It is recommended for improving day-to-day concentration and attention, and encourages calmness and serenity as you practise, at any time of day.

Today we are going to spend the day with our friend the flamingo. Let's imitate them!

1. The flamingo

Put your weight on your left foot, and lift your right foot and place it behind your left calf.

Keep your balance in this pose and then lift your arms up and out by your sides, to open up the flamingo's wings.

If you can balance well enough, try to take off by flapping your arms up and down. Then change legs.

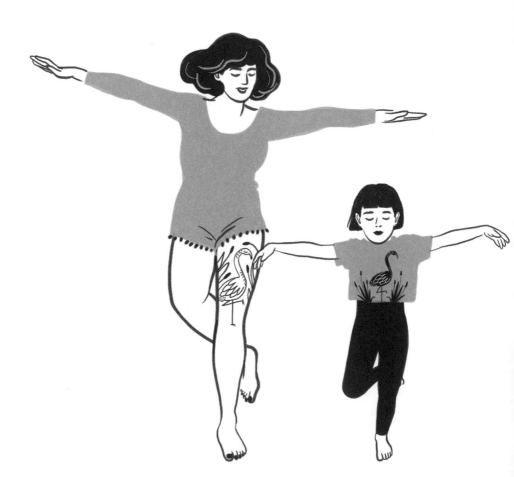

The flamingos spend some time in the forest and go to see their favourite tree.

2. The flamingo's favourite tree

Stand with your weight on your right foot and your left foot on the calf or thigh of your right leg.

Your right leg should be straight, stable and anchored to the floor, like the trunk of a tree. Your left foot should be carefully planted on your right leg, like a branch of the tree.

Lift both hands towards the sky as if they were two more branches.

Stay balanced in this position and breathe deeply.

If you are comfortable like this, you can move your arms as if they were branches moving in the wind.

Then put your left foot back on the floor and change sides.

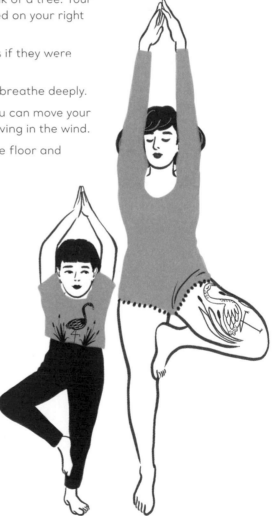

Do not put your foot on the other knee, as that is a joint and if you press too hard it could be painful! To have a bit of fun, you can get into tree pose and ask your child to test your stability by tickling you! However, you'll get to swap roles afterwards.

The flamingo is going to collect itself next to a very impressive tree.

3. The mightiest tree in the forest

It's the same principle as the previous tree, but this time in a pair!

Stand side by side, holding on to each other, either by the waist or by the shoulder and leg for little ones. Make a trunk with two legs together and make the branches of the tree: one of you places their right foot on their left leg and the other places their left foot on the right leg.

Each of you lifts your outer arms to make two more branches of the tree.

Breathe as you hold this position, keep your balance together and then change sides.

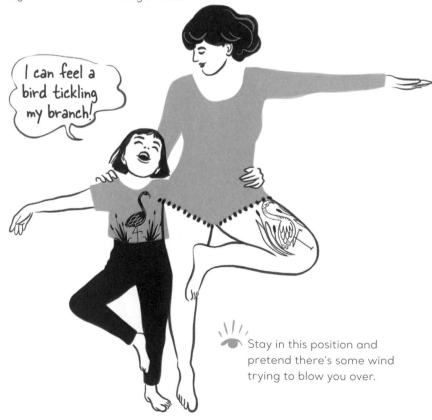

I can feel a bird tickling my branch!

Stay in this position and pretend there's some wind trying to blow you over.

The flamingo stretches its wings and flies over a palm grove.

4. The palm tree

Stand facing each other with your feet hip-width apart.

Stand up on tiptoes and reach up with your hands, keeping fingers straight. Try to touch the sky!

Keep balancing on your tiptoes, then bend your knees to get as low as you can. If you can, crouch down, keeping your hands straight up.

Then start again with your feet together.

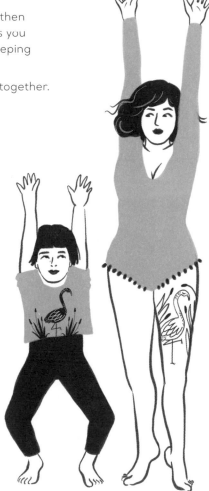

As it flies, the flamingo comes across a magnificent eagle.

5. The eagle

Stand with your weight on your left foot and bend your left knee to let your right leg wrap around the left, so one thigh is crossed over.

If you can, curl your right foot around your left calf.

Lift your arms out by your sides to make big eagle wings and fly!

As you breathe in, lift your arms up and as you breathe out lower them.

Then change legs.

 If you want to, and your balance permits, you can try out a more difficult pose. When you're standing on your left leg, hold your right arm bent in front of you and curl your left arm around it so your hands meet in front of your face. Use your arms and legs to stay stable while you try to keep your elbows and knees in the same line!

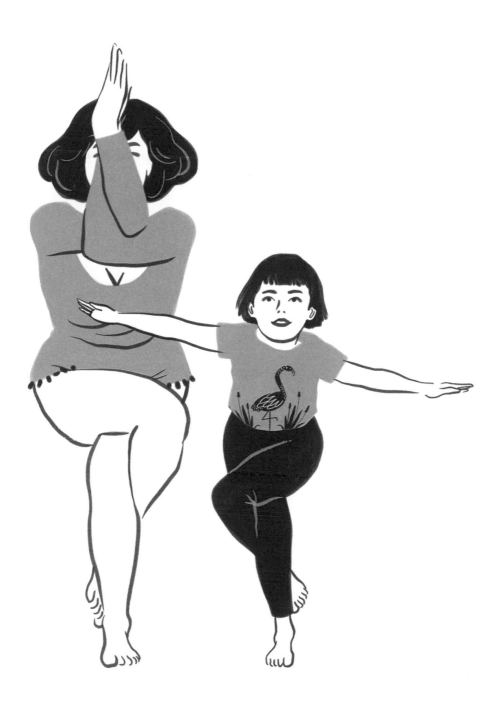

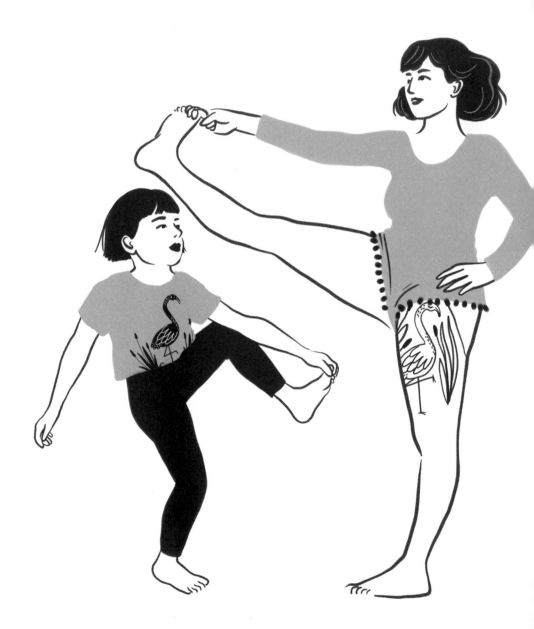

After a long flight, the flamingo needs to do a few exercises to stretch its legs.

6. The leg game

Stand with your weight on your left leg and hold your right knee at chest level with both hands, breathing and keeping your balance.

Either place your hands beneath your right knee or hold your right big toe with your index finger, middle finger and thumb of your right hand. Then straighten your right leg in front of you. Try to touch your partner's foot while you keep your balance.

Bring your right knee back to your chest and change sides.

 Try to gauge the correct distance between the two of you at the start so you can touch your feet together without moving around while you get into the pose.

Now do the same thing to the side.

Standing with your weight on your left leg, bend your right knee and bring it up to your right side. Then either place your right hand under the knee or grip your big toe with your index finger, middle finger and thumb.

Gently straighten your leg to the right and hold your left arm out to the left in order to keep your balance.

Then bend your leg again and change sides.

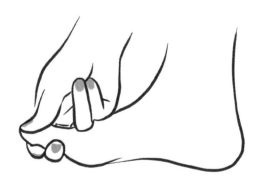

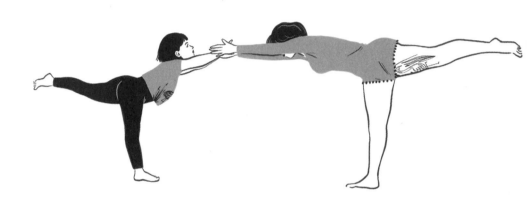

7. The warrior 3

Stand facing each other and, with your arms out, hold each
other's hands.

Stand with your weight on your straight right leg, and slowly lift
your left leg up behind you. If you can, try and get it level with
your hips.

Your toes and knee should be facing the floor, your left leg and
arms should be straight. Your body should be parallel to the floor,
so tilt the left side of your hips towards the floor.

Breathe as you hold the pose and replace your left leg before
changing sides.

Now that it has done some exercises, the flamingo goes back to its friends and is keen to show off how supple it is now. It is ready to show its friends what it can do.

8. Supple like a flamingo

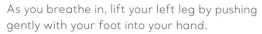

Face each other, put your weight on your right leg, bend your left knee and grasp the inside of your left foot with your left hand behind your body.

Hold on to each other with your right hand straight out in front of you.

As you breathe in, lift your left leg by pushing gently with your foot into your hand.

Gradually lift up higher in your own time, without letting your body lean forwards. Keep your torso as straight as possible without straining.

Breathe as you hold the pose. Then, as you breathe out, place your left foot back down and change sides.

To finish the demonstration, the flamingo makes a surprising bow to its applauding friends.

9. The flamingo's bow

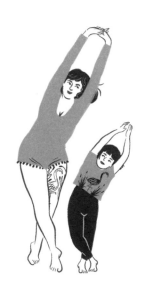

Facing each other, cross your right leg in front of your left leg and lift your hands above your head. Then lean over to your left side to stretch your right side.

Breathe for a few cycles as you stretch deeply, then slowly come back to centre before changing sides.

After a lovely day, it's time for the flamingo to go home and sit down comfortably in its chair.

10. The flamingo in its chair

Stand up facing each other with your feet slightly apart and hold hands.

Breathe in, bend your knees and move down as if you were going to sit in a chair.

Breathe as you hold this pose. As you breathe out, come back up slowly.

Repeat the exercise with your feet together.

Then turn back to back, slowly move downwards to a seated position and carry on going down until you are in yogi pose.

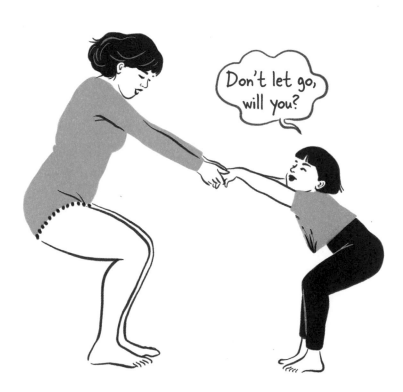

Before going to bed, the flamingo plays with its child.
They invent the game of roly-poly flamingos.

11. Roly-poly flamingos

In back to back yogi pose, wrap your elbows around each other's
and shift your weight back and forth with your backs together.

One of you should curl forwards and the other open out their
back by leaning backwards. Then do the opposite.

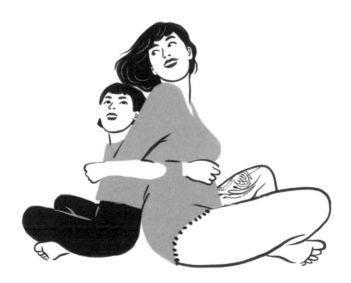

12. Relaxation

And now for some relaxation!

Lie down in whatever position feels comfortable
(for guided relaxation, see page 28).

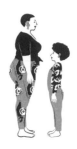 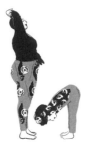 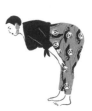 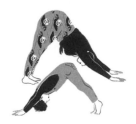

1. The mountain   2. Coming down the mountain   3. Right angle   4. Downward-facing dog

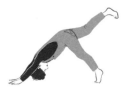 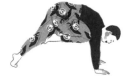 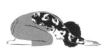

5. Downward-facing dog with a leg out   6. Downward-facing dog with a paw under its chest   7. Child's pose

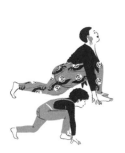 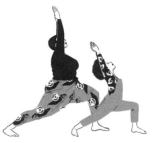 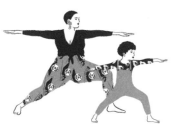

8. Warrior on one knee   9. The warrior 1   10. The warrior 2

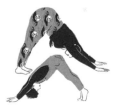 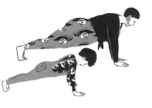 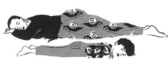

11. Downward-facing dog   12. The plank   13. Flat-as-a-pancake relaxation

Warrior training

For all ages
Advanced level
For any time of day, apart from evening
Duration: 25 to 30 minutes

This session is for you and your child if your child has practised yoga a few times before.

It's good for when they need to let off steam, channel their energy or when they're feeling angry.

This is a good sequence for reinforcing the muscles of the back and the abdominal wall.

However, it is dynamic and therefore not recommended for the evening.

To start our training, the warriors are going to imitate a majestic mountain.

1. The mountain

Stand up straight face to face, feet together with your big toes touching.

Make sure you stand up really tall, legs and arms straight, to create a really nice mountain.

Take a big deep breath and breathe out in a deep, fluid manner.

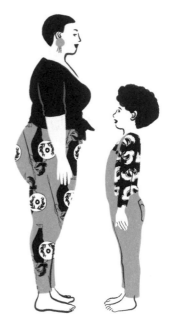

2. Coming down the mountain

Grasp your elbows behind your head and stretch upwards. From this position, lower your body slowly, keeping your back straight, and at the end of the movement put your hands near to your feet.

Your legs don't need to be tense and it shouldn't strain your lower back. If it does, bend your knees a little so you're in a comfortable position for the whole lowering movement.

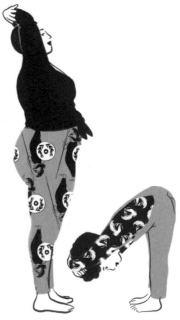

The next exercise is to strengthen the warrior's back and stomach muscles.

3. Right angle

From the coming down the mountain pose, stay leaning forward and widen your stance a little. Breathe in, put your hands on your calves or your thighs and, as you breathe out, bring your back parallel to the floor, making sure you have a good back stretch.

Try to get your heads closer to each other, but make sure you don't arch or round your back!

Breathe deeply in this position, making sure you keep your back as straight as possible.

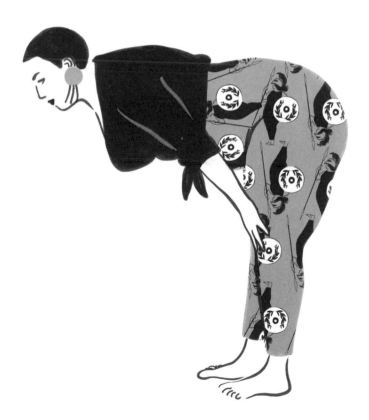

4. Downward-facing dog

Get on to all fours. Place your hands on the floor at the front of your mat and take a big step backwards to put first one foot and then the other to the back of your mat.

Breathe in and push your hands so you lift your hips towards the sky. Make an upside-down V with your body.

Your hands should be shoulder-width apart, fingers spread out and pointing to the front. Your knees should be hip-width apart.

Push hard with your hands, keeping your shoulders relaxed and your head tucked in. Look at your belly button.

To start with, keep your toes on the floor. Then bend your right knee and stretch out your left leg by putting your left heel on the floor. Then do the same on the other side.

Alternate between the sides. If you can, get both of your heels on the floor.

In this pose, have some fun by each going underneath the downward-facing dog, making sure there is enough space between hands and feet, and between hips and floor!

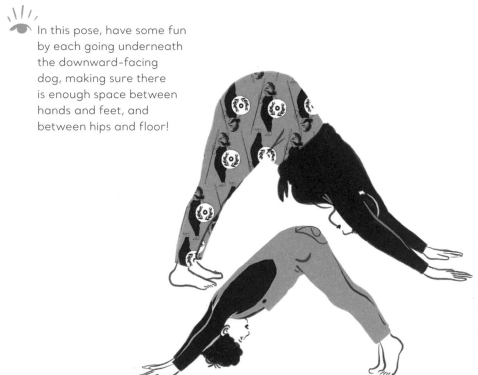

5. Downward-facing dog with a leg out

When you are in downward-facing dog pose, breathe in.

When you breathe out, lift your right leg upwards to stretch your right hip.

Then, keeping your leg in the air, bend your knee so your right foot goes towards your left. This will cause a deeper stretch in your right hip, as well as your right side.

Breathe in, place your foot back on the mat and repeat on the other side. Do this twice on each side.

Your hands should be well anchored to the floor and the foot on the floor should be stable too. You should look towards your feet or, for the more advanced, in the direction of your left armpit, as if you were looking at your right foot when the knee is bent.

6. Downward-facing dog with a paw under its chest

Go back to the downward-facing dog pose and, as you breathe in, bring your right knee in towards your belly button by rounding your back.

Breathe out. Then put your right foot back behind you on the mat and repeat the movement with your left foot.

Repeat this four times on each side.

If you're comfortable, stay in this pose and do a few quick breaths in and out.

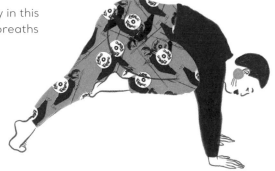

Now it's time for the warriors to have a little rest: store up some energy for the remainder of the session.

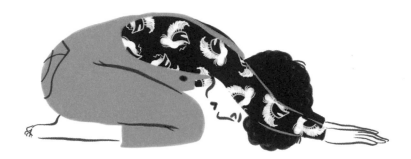

7. Child's pose

After the downward-facing dog pose, breathe in, bend your knees and, as you breathe out, sit down on your heels with your feet together, knees slightly apart.

Lower your chest down to the floor or a cushion if it's more comfortable.

Keep your arms out in front of you, elbows on the floor, hands pointing in the direction of the front of your mat. Relax into this pose, breathing deeply a few times.

The warriors can now try out their legendary strength in different poses.

8. Warrior on one knee

From the child's pose, breathe in and get into downward-facing dog pose (see 4, page 224).

Without moving your hands, breathe out and bring your right foot forwards between your hands, then lower your left knee to the floor.

Keep your knee on the floor and your hands in position. Straighten up your ribcage and look straight in front of you as you breathe in.

When you breathe out, come back to downward-facing dog pose and then do the same movement with the other leg.

If this pose is comfortable and stable, stretch your arms upwards above your head and look up.

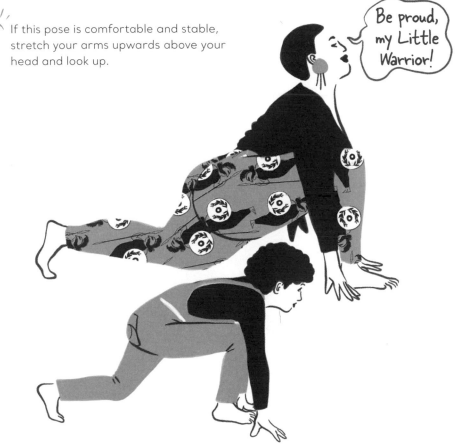

Be proud, my Little Warrior!

9. The warrior 1

Facing each other in the downward-facing dog pose, place your left foot between your hands with your knee bent.

Keep your chest straight and facing in the direction of the front of the mat.

Put your right foot at a 45-degree angle to the heel of your left foot, toes towards the front, and turn your hips to face the front of the mat.

Bend your left knee so it's directly above your left ankle and keep your right leg straight. Raise your arms.

Then look at each other and hold out your arms towards each other to share your warrior strength.

Go back to downward-facing dog pose and change sides.

You can stretch and bend the front leg, gently pushing and pulling on each other's hands, to make a more dynamic pose.

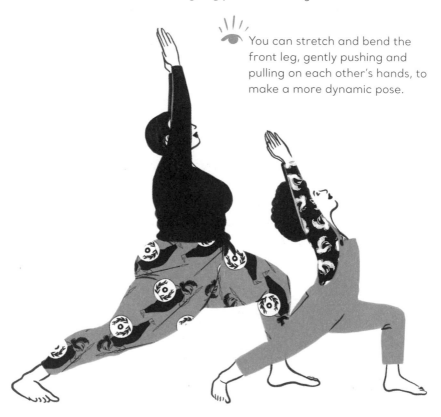

10. The warrior 2

From the downward-facing dog pose, breathe in and place your left foot between your hands with your knee bent. Breathe out and bring your torso up.

Turn your hips and torso to face the long side of your mat.

Your right leg should be at a 90-degree angle to the heel of your left foot (that's the one in front) and your right toes should face the direction of the long part of the mat.

Bend your left knee so it is directly over your left ankle. Your right leg should be straight.

Lift your arms up straight to shoulder height and hold hands in front to share your warrior strength.

Breathe deeply and find a stable, comfortable position.

Then go back to downward-facing dog and change sides.

If you try this facing each other, you can stretch and bend the front leg, gently pushing and pulling on each other's hand to make a more dynamic pose.

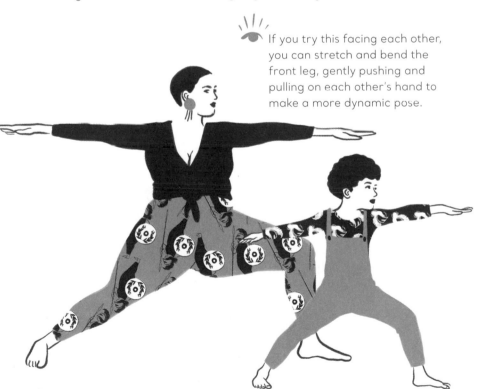

11. Downward-facing dog

Breathe in and out a few times in downward-facing dog pose.

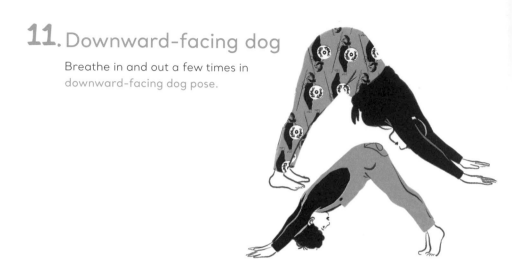

Time for the final exercise in the warrior's training.

12. The plank

From the downward-facing dog pose, breathe out and move your ribcage so it's parallel to the floor. Tuck your chin in.

Keep both arms and legs straight, and place both feet together at the back of your mat. Keep your head straight at the top of your shoulders. Your body should be in a straight line from your neck to your feet.

Use your breathing to stay in this position by inhaling and exhaling deeply.

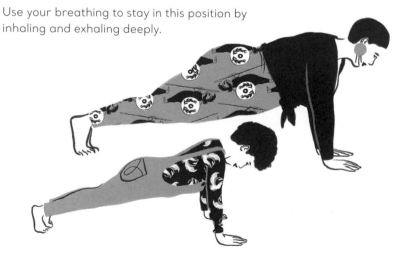

That's it! The warriors have passed their training, so it's time for a well-earned rest.

13. Flat-as-a-pancake relaxation

From the plank pose, lie down on your front in a comfortable position.

And now for some relaxation (for guided relaxation, see page 28).

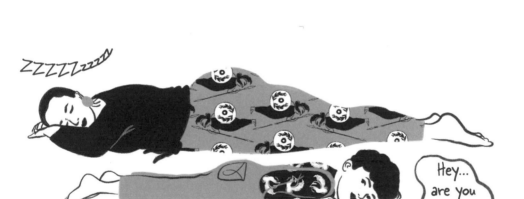

ZZZZZzzz

Hey... are you sleeping?

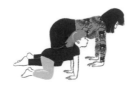
1. Wrist warm-up

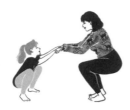
2. Pushing on hands and fingers

3. Monkey walking on the floor

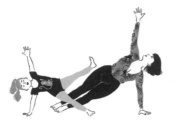
4. Monkey plank

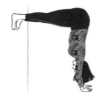
5. Monkey's yogi squat

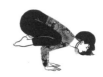
6. The crow

7. Monkey's upside-down pyramid

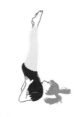
8. Monkey walks up the wall with their feet

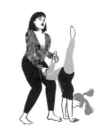
9. Monkey balance

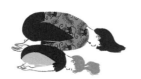
10. Child's pose

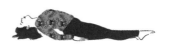
11. The candle

12. The fish

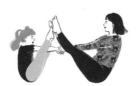
13. Boat on the water

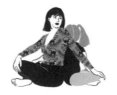
14. Seated back-to-back twists

15. Relaxation

The monkey

For all ages
Advanced level
For any time of day, apart from evening
Duration: 20 to 25 minutes

This is a dynamic sequence for the morning or afternoon.
It can help to improve motor skills and concentration in very
young children (and adults), as well as self-confidence.
Pregnant women or women at the start of their menstrual
cycle shouldn't attempt this sequence, as there are many
inverted poses, which are not recommended.

Monkeys are very agile animals and they love to have fun. Let's do what they do!
Can you imitate a monkey? How do they move?
How do they sound?
In order to behave like monkeys, we're going to warm up and strengthen our wrists.

1. Wrist warm-up

Sit down in yogi pose.

Your elbows should be next to your body and your hands in front of you.

Put your hand together, cross your fingers and make circular movements with your wrists, first one way, then the other.

While you warm up, keep your back straight and breathe deeply.

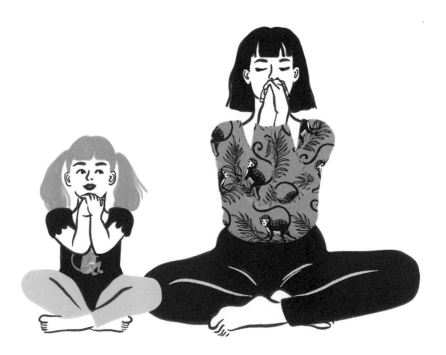

2. Pushing on hands and fingers

Get on to all fours and press down on your hands. Feel your fingers anchored to the floor one by one, then spread your fingers out and press down on all of them again, one by one.

Place your hands on the floor in front of you, then to one side and then the other, then with fingers towards you, and, finally, with the backs of your hands on the floor, to stretch out all around your wrists and forearms.

Along with your child, assign a number to each finger so you can keep track of which ones you are pressing with.

Now our wrists are ready, we can move around like monkeys.

3. Monkey walking on the floor

Crouch down and move around the room using your hands in the way monkeys do. Have fun! You can put all your weight on your hands to raise your hips and move around like this on one side and then the other.

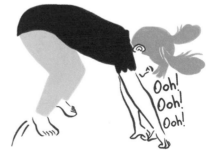

Ooh! Ooh! Ooh!

Monkeys need very strong arms and legs to move from tree to tree in the Amazon forest. We are going to have some fun using ours to become as agile as them!

4. Monkey plank

Leaning on your hands, make your ribcage parallel to the floor by bringing your chin in and keep both arms straight. Then move both feet to the back of your mat and straighten your legs.

Make a straight plank without arching your back. Use your breathing to help you stay in this position by breathing in and out deeply.

Now do a plank with one less element.

Shift your body weight to the right side and lift up your left hand. Then do the same on the other side by lifting your right hand. Then make it even better by lifting one leg and then the other!

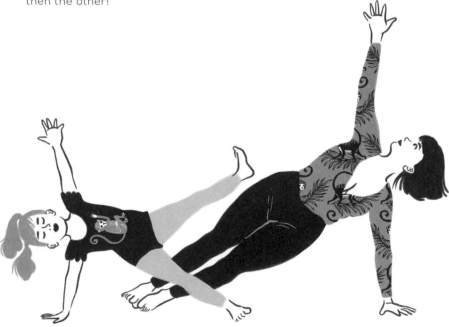

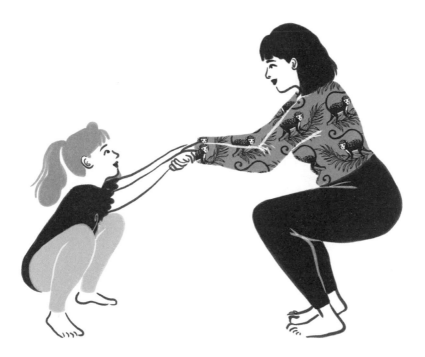

5. Monkey's yogi squat

Crouch down facing each other and hold each other's hands.

Work together to balance, keeping your feet apart and, if possible, your heels on the floor.

This exercise is often easier for children than it is for parents.

Find the leg distance that works best for you: some people find yogi squats easy with their feet together, others don't. Everyone has a different level of flexibility. Once you have both found a comfortable pose, test out how effective it is by letting go of each other's hands. If you fall over, start again!

6. The crow

Crouch down in the yogi squat position (5) with your feet wide apart.

Put your hands down flat in front of you, fingers spread out and anchored on the floor. Lift as high as you can on your toes. Bend your elbows into your inside leg.

Place one bent knee on one arm almost at your armpit and then, taking your time, do the same on the other side.

Try one side, then the other, to find out which is the easiest and most comfortable for you.

When you have one knee in place, move the second one slowly.

Make sure your toes are still touching the floor and look straight in front of you to keep your balance.

Tense your abs and push into the floor with your hands to help you lift first one foot, then the other, and to hold the pose.

This is not an easy pose. Try it a few times keeping one foot on the floor to make it less challenging.

👁 Help your child by placing yourself behind them, so that you can hold one of their legs and show them whereabouts on the upper arm to place their knee.

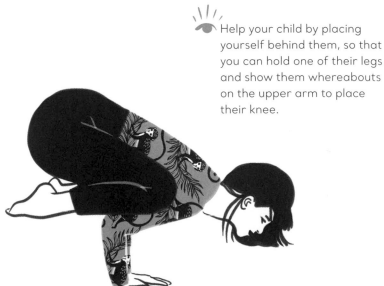

We have done a lot of work on our arms and legs. Now let's play around with our heads down and our feet in the air, like monkeys when they have fun hanging from trees.

7. Monkey's upside-down pyramid

Get down on your knees. Sit on your heels and put your hands flat on the floor in front of your knees.

Imagine a triangle. Its baseline goes between your two hands. The top is the point on the floor where you will place your head.

Put your head on the mat and bend your elbows, your arms parallel to the floor.

Gently place one knee on one arm. Then, when you're comfortable, place the other knee on the other arm.

Push into the ground with your hands and slowly lift your hips towards the sky.

Keep your shoulders away from your ears to make yourself bigger and to get greater stability in your upside-down pyramid.

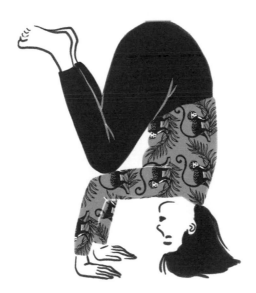

8. Monkey walks up the wall with their feet

Get into downward-facing dog pose (see page 50), but with your heels against a wall that you will be able to put your feet against as you stand on your hands.

Get into a stable position on your two hands and lift one foot and place it against the wall. Then raise your hips and place the other foot on the wall.

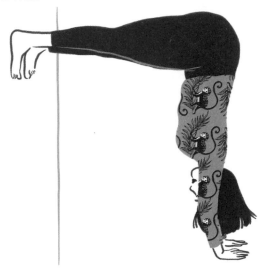

In your own time, move your feet higher and higher, and move your hands closer to the wall in order to balance with your legs in the air. Always keep your feet on the wall.

 It's a good idea to show your child this pose first, so they can imitate you.

The first time they do it, guide your child into the pose safely. To do this, you could hold their hips or help them to place their feet on the wall one by one.

For very small children, don't use a wall. Instead, sit down and suggest your child gets into downward-facing dog pose with their heels towards you. They can put their feet on your knees. Then if they're comfortable with the pressure on their hands, they can put their feet on your shoulders.

9. Monkey balance

This pose is recommended for children who are comfortable with supporting their weight on their hands, but they will need your help.

Stand beside your child. get them to place their hands on the floor and then put one, then the other, leg up, in order to balance.

To be comfortable and stable in this position, your child should tense their abs, keep their shoulders away from their ears to make their body as long as they can, and keep their back as straight as possible.

You can hold your child's feet to help them push their arms as much as possible and to make sure they don't curve their back too much. In this pose your body should be like a straight line and not a banana!

Once your child is comfortable getting in to this pose by themselves you can do it together.

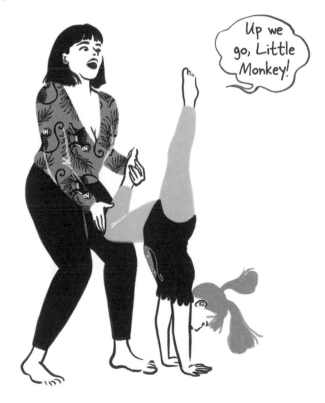

The monkey needs some rest after all those upside-down poses – and so do we!

10. Child's pose

Get on your knees and sit down on your heels. Lean forwards until your forehead touches the floor. Your arms should be next to your body, palms facing upwards.

Stay in this pose for a while to relax and breathe deeply.

To move out of this pose, put your hands under your shoulders and uncurl your back gently, starting with your lower back. Your head should come up last.

If, when you lean forwards, you or your child don't touch the floor with your forehead, you can put down a cushion (or two) and rest your head on it.

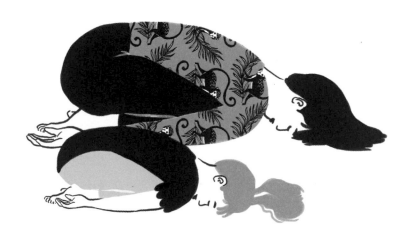

Now that we've got some energy back, let's have some fun with our legs in the air.

11. The candle

Lie on your back with your arms beside your body, palms down.

Raise your legs to 90 degrees from the floor.

Lift your pelvis up to get into candle pose. Put your hands on your lower back, elbows on the floor.

Take long, deep breaths to help you stay in this position.

For the youngest children, or those who aren't used to this pose, help them at first by lifting their legs and holding them as straight as possible. Also help them to get out of this position by carefully unrolling their back.

Women shouldn't do this pose if they are pregnant or at the start of their menstrual cycle.

Next, gently move your straight legs behind your head.

Stay in this position and, if you can, put your toes on the floor. Breathe.

Then, staying in this pose, spread your legs. Breathe.

Bring your legs back together and bend your knees in order to get them as close as you can to your ears.

To get out of this position, keep your knees bent and gently bring your legs back in front of you. Stay lying down for a little while.

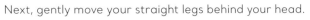
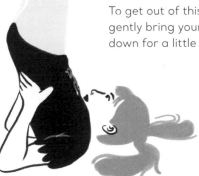

Next to the forest there is a river. We can see some fish swimming upside-down for fun. Let's do as they do!

12. The fish

Lying on your back, put your head at the front of your mat.

With your legs straight and feet together, place your arms beside your body with your palms facing downwards.

Breathe in and bend your elbows in order to lift your upper body.

Gently tip your head backwards and put the top of your head on the floor. Look at you with your head upside down!

Then, lifting your head up first, bring your body back to the floor.

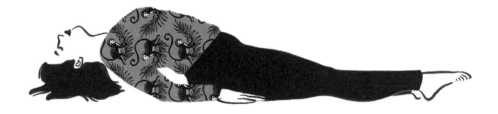

This pose opens up the ribcage. Don't force it, do it progressively. There shouldn't be any pain in your neck. If your head doesn't touch the floor, place a cushion down so that you are in a comfortable position.

There is a boat on the river. Let's get in and go for a row!

13. Boat on the water

Sit down facing each other. With your legs apart flat on the floor, put your feet together and hold each other's hands.

To row the boat, take turns to pull the other one forward, trying to reach as far as possible.

Continue this forwards and backwards movement and lean to the right. Come back to the centre and then lean to the left. Continue like this, but be careful not to fall in the water!

Still facing each other, get a bit closer and put your feet together, knees bent upwards, and hold hands.

Then lift your feet up together as high as you can, inside your joined arms. Hold this position. Then try the same position lifting your feet up on the outside of your arms. Continue to raise your feet inside and outside, but – again – don't fall in the water!

For the second part of the boat trip, you can lift just one foot, then the other, until you get your balance and are able to lift both at the same time.

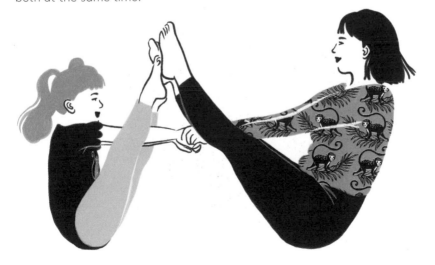

We have returned from a lovely boat trip and now we're going to relax our backs.

14. Seated back-to-back twists

Sit back to back in yogi pose.

Twist around with your upper back. As you breathe in, grasp your left knee with your right hand and with your left hand grasp your partner's knee. Breathe as you twist.

As you breathe out, come back to the centre. Breathe in and change sides.

Your head should follow the movement of your back. Your back should be like a pearl necklace that rolls around one way then the other in fluid fashion.

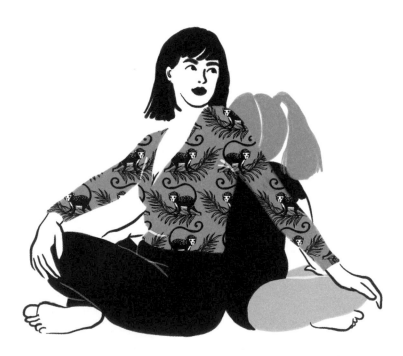

15. Relaxation

And now for some relaxation (for guided relaxation, see page 28).

Index

Sessions in alphabetical order

butterfly, The	91
camel, The	189
cat, The	53
duck, The	155
elephant, The	141
fairy, The	121
flamingo's day, The	207
grasshopper, The	173
introduction to the joints of your body, An	37
koala, The	63
monkey, The	233
strange magic machine, The	75
walk by the pond, A	103
Sun salutation	45
Warrior training	221

Sessions by time of day

Sessions for any time of day

An introduction to the joints of your body   37

The strange magic machine   75

The butterfly   91

The flamingo's day   207

Dynamic sessions (morning or afternoon, not evening)

Sun salutation   45

A walk by the pond   103

The fairy   121

The elephant   141

The duck   155

The grasshopper   173

The camel   189

Warrior training   221

The monkey   233

Relaxing sessions (perfect for evening, or any time of day)

The cat   53

The koala   63

Sessions by length of time

5–15/20 minutes

An introduction to the joints of your body   37

Sun salutation   45

10–15 minutes

The cat   53

15–20 minutes

The koala   63

The strange magic machine   75

The butterfly   91

The flamingo's day   207

20–25 minutes

The elephant   141

The duck   155

The monkey   233

25–30 minutes

A walk by the pond   103

The fairy   121

The grasshopper   173

The camel   189

Warrior training   221

Notes

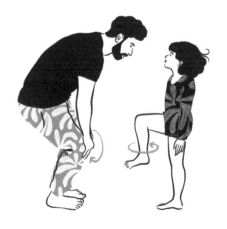

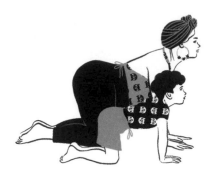

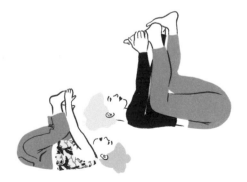